I0058045

Stem Cell 101:
Demystify Your Medicine of the Future

Stem Cell 101:
Demystify Your Medicine of the Future

Tony V. Lu, M.D.

Stem Cell 101:
Demystify Your Medicine of the Future

Copyright © 2014
by Tony V. Lu, M.D.

Cover design by Lucy Swerdfeger

All rights reserved. No part of this book may be used or reproduced in any matter whatsoever with out written permission from the Publisher, except in the case of brief quotations embodied in articles and reviews.

Published by
NEW MEDICINE PRESS
Scottsdale, Arizona

ISBN information

Paperback — 978-1-93842-76-0 — $ 14.95

e-Book — 978-1-932842-77-7 — $ 9.99

www.NewMedicinePress.com

Printed in the United States of America

Table of Contents

We are born full of curiosity.
When something is good, we long to make it better.
When something is broken, we aim to fix it.

This book is dedicated to all who explore the unknown
and who are gifted in asking the next question as
they search to improve the universe.

octors and scientists *live* for Eureka moments — those exhilarating times when our ideas are proven sound and we are ready to bring life-altering innovation into the world. Like so many others, I grew up idolizing the men and women who made history in the close quarters of the research laboratory – renowned scientists who halted deadly diseases and gave us far-reaching cures. For those not familiar with the path of scientific exploration, let me clue you in on an inside secret. Few discoveries are at once iconic. Doctors and scientists know that our best moments are more likely to be just small steps — hopefully important steps — along the way to something greater. One Eureka moment paves the way for another.

This is the way research works, especially in the world of stem cells.

There have been sensational discoveries, perhaps none more so than the creation of *Dolly*, the world's first cloned mammal; a feat that was made possible only after twentieth-century scientists understood the nature of stem cells. Even more amazing, once cloned, Dolly's mere existence forced the scientific community, but also religious and political leaders, to come to terms with the definition of our humanity. Would we, as mankind, consent to the cloning of a human being?

Fortunately, credible scientists tend to agree: cloning for reproductive purposes doesn't sit well with us, just as it doesn't with the conscientious-thinking public. There is no good reason to clone a total and an exact replica of ourselves as a shrine to human existence. The real value of stem cell research lies in the ability to cure and prevent diseases; to make living healthier and more comfortable.

During the writing of this book, two esteemed researchers joined the ranks of the science rock stars; they have earned the right to be included in the same breath as Jonas Salk, who created the polio vaccine, and Alexander Fleming, who created penicillin. In 2012, John B. Gurdon and Shinya Yamanaka were jointly honored with the Nobel Prize in Physiology or Medicine for their revelations in stem cell possibilities. Gurdon and Yamanaka, the latter building on the discovery of the former forty years earlier, challenged the way scientists understood the development of specialized cells. The two proved that specialized cells could be reprogrammed and function as other cells of the body, paving the way for real hope in curing disease. These specialized cells are called stem cells.

Now that stem cell research has been given its respectable due by those in the Nobel community, it follows that greater public acceptance is likely to occur. The thing is, some of the old perceptions about stem cell research no longer fit the twenty-first century, where the population is aging and more people are susceptible to serious, often no-hope diseases — and are in need of a cure. Where once research was based on the modification of *embryonic* stem cells, today's advancements are more likely to involve *adult* stem cells that are as accessible as human skin — where fetuses are never touched. Thanks to the discoveries of Nobel winners Gurdon and Yamanaka, other scientists are embarking on their own Eureka journeys, moving closer to curing cancer and other aging diseases like heart disease and Parkinson's. Researchers offer new hope for children too, including those born with diabetes and autism.

Will stem cells provide the ultimate Eureka answers? They just might. Here are 101 important questions about stem cells — and 101 easy to understand answers.

— Tony V. Lu, M.D.

Chapter 1

Fearing the Unknown:
Why are Some People so Afraid
of Stem Cell Research?

efore we look at more serious objections to stem cell research, it is worth noting how closely related science and science fiction are. Could our earliest fears have been formed on a Saturday afternoon in childhood as we watched scary black & white monster movies?

Our earliest Frankensteins plotted to control the world. They harmed man. They were born (thankfully only in fiction) from scientific experiments gone astray or were purposely conceived in a lab by a villain to do his dirty work. Some people have insisted that if this abuse of science, nature, and power could happen in the movies, it could happen in real life. They fear that stem cell research might lead to the unnatural process of cloning a human being; and that these technologies could fall into the hands of the wrong people who would create submissive armies of humans for their own rewards. For some people, *stem cells* are *scary* because they seem much like the evil in a Frankenstein nightmare.

Of course, there have been other reasons people have feared stem cell research; some have a mistrust of government policies that fund much of our scientific medical research. Historically, experimentation has been conducted on vulnerable segments of society, including the mentally ill, prisoners, and impoverished people. Certain racial populations have also been major participants in these research pools.

1

What Happened in Alabama?

In 1932, the Tuskegee Institute of Alabama originated a study to determine the long term effects of venereal disease on the body. It enlisted 600 men from the region's African American community — 399 with syphilis and 201 who were syphilis-free to be used as the control group. In return for participating in the publicly funded study, the men were given free food and medical exams along with treatments containing heavy metals such as neoarsephenamine, bismuth, and mercury, as well as over-the-counter medications like aspirin. Crude as it was, it was ongoing treatment that the participants could not afford otherwise. When the men underwent more complex diagnosing (including a spinal tap), it was likely for the benefit of the study rather than for the patients' well being. Doctors believed that the biggest contribution these men would make toward the understanding of syphilis would occur after the death of the patients, so the men were also given burial insurance on the condition that an autopsy was performed.

Over the course of their care, these men were not adequately briefed about their health; in fact, they were not aware that they were being treated for syphilis. They were only informed that they had *bad blood,* a general description of the times that encompassed a number of illnesses including syphilis, anemia, and fatigue. Even after penicillin was commonly recognized as a treatment for syphilis, the men were not given the drug, nor were they given the option of withdrawing from the study. Forty years later the study was deemed unjustified. It was halted in 1972 and in 1974 a $10 million dollar out-of-court settlement was reached with the men and their families.

Today the Tuskegee Syphilis Study is viewed as one of medicine's most unethical government-funded research studies.

Two decades after the Tuskegee study began, a Maryland researcher at Johns Hopkins Hospital biopsied tissue taken from a woman with a cervical cancer tumor and cultivated it in a petri dish. What he found in the tissue were identified as the world's first known immortal cells — cells that could divide and live indefinitely. Technically, these cells were not stem cells because they failed to meet a key requirement: they did not repair themselves or the body. Still, these rare cells taught researchers much about the nature of stem cells and this cell line continues to be medically useful today. These cells are known as HeLa cells, a coded variation for the Baltimore patient's name, Henrietta Lacks.

In 1951, Henrietta was a poor tobacco farmer in Virginia who sought treatment in Hopkins' indigent care clinic. It was customary then (as it is today) for biopsied tissue, organs, and other parts removed from the body to be considered medical waste and not the property of the patient. Traditionally, medical researchers have used this "waste" for study and experimentation — just as they were used in Henrietta's case. Her immortal cells, however, were unique. As her cancer cells divided and the quantity grew, the cells were collected in a cell bank.

HeLa cells have had far-reaching impact in many areas of scientific study. They have been essential in the development of the polio vaccine. They've been to the moon to measure the effects of gravity on cancer, and they have had an important role in discoveries pertaining to cloning, gene-mapping, and in-vitro fertilization. To conduct this research, as well as federally funded studies found in hospitals around the world, HeLa cells have been marketed and sold from the cell bank to other researchers, creating a billion dollar industry. Henrietta never received compensation for her monumental contribution to science. Ironically, she and her family relied on indigent medical care for the remainder of their lives. Although researchers at Hopkins did nothing illegal in marketing Henrietta's cells, nor did they adhere to devious or unethical medical practices in obtaining them, Hopkins earned a great deal of money from these cells, all the while those who were the source of their good fortune remained in such poverty. Viewed from outside the medical profession, this inequity seems grossly unfair. HeLa cells became more than medical resources, they became *Big Business*.

The mistrust of Big Business is yet another reason some people have been apprehensive about stem cell research.

What Will Happen when Stem Cell Research Becomes the Stem Cell Industry?

Consider the controversy involving genetically-altered seed that began with farmers in small rural communities but reached the heights of the 1980 United States Supreme Court. The Monsanto firm, a corporate leader in the areas of agriculture and biotechnology, conducted DNA studies that resulted in new types of hybrid seed that produced not only bigger yields, but crops that were more resistant to weather and disease. Of course the farmers benefitted from these newly genetically-altered seeds and they liked planting them, until Monsanto accused many of them of violating product rights and threatened them with legal action. By 2006, nearly 2,400 farmers in 19 states were investigated for rights infringements. Monsanto would later emphasize that during a 15-year period, only 145 lawsuits were actually filed and only nine of these had gone to trial. The company admitted though that nearly 700 matters had been settled out of court.

These product infringements centered on a time-honored practice in the farming industry. Traditionally, as farmers harvested their crops, they also harvested the newly formed seed generated by those crops, collecting it for their next planting cycle. Not only was this good crop management, it also reduced the amount of seed they needed for the next planting. However, having patented the hybrid seed, Monsanto now controlled its destiny.

At one point, the Center for Food Safety in Washington, DC estimated that Monsanto employed 75 individuals armed with a $10 million dollar annual budget to prosecute farmers who were replanting the hybrid seed, thereby cutting into Monsanto's profits. The company was accused of going further still, incriminating farmers who had never planted the hybrid seed in the first place, but who had come by the plants unintentionally.

As wind and the weather descended upon the hybrid seed, nature swept it into the fields of the neighborhood farmers. According to one testimony, when Monsanto agents scoured these fields for even the

4

smallest traces of the renegade seed *and found it*, they slapped lawsuits upon these farmers as well, although farmers insisted that had not planted the Monsanto product. The legal fees for defending their positions, both real and perceived, forced many farmers out of business. Meanwhile, the farm community abruptly discovered that it had lost a great deal of both ownership and control over crops cultivated on its own farmland. The patent on this hybrid seed is set to expire in 2014, allowing other seed companies to manufacture their own hybrid versions and market them to the farmers. However, there have also been complaints by farmers that Monsanto has been pressuring them to contract for the next generation of Monsanto hybrid seed. In obtaining these contracts, the company will once again have significant control over the farmers' yields.

Will medical procedures derived from gene-altered stem cells follow the same course of the Monsanto gene-altered seed? Will the value of stem cells become more about profit and control than saving patients? Many feel that the act of saving someone's life should be above this.

Does Controversy Make for Better Decisions?

Perhaps nothing has deterred the advancement of stem cell research in the United States more than the stance taken by conservative groups who have been determined to halt stem cell experimentation. Some have done so out of personal religious beliefs, but many remain involved for political gain. By aligning embryonic stem cell research with the issue of abortion, ultra conservatives equated the death of a cell with the death of a fetus or human life. Although not all in their political party or their religious affiliations subscribed to the narrow definition of *life* that allowed conservatives to make such an accusation, the outcry was loud and forceful enough to derail legal status for future experimentation on a wide scale, and once the legality of experimentation was in question, funding sources for the projects dried up.

When Japanese scientist Shinya Yamanaka succeeded in reprogramming adult stem cells to near-embryonic status in 2006, researchers believed they now had the viable new source they needed to begin future experimentation — without the legal threats caused by the *embryonic* stem cell controversy. In adult reprogrammed stem cells, researchers had gained the ability to study human cell development from its earliest stage to old age. It opened the door for the examination of disease at its onset. In time, scientists hope to reprogram diseased cells back to their healthy state. What a boon this would be for medical advancements!

***

When race, vulnerability, and medical ethics — not to mention politics, money, and power — all come into play, it is easy to understand why people might be apprehensive about stem cell experimentation. Should researchers give into the fears of some and never attempt to go forward with groundbreaking innovation that could save the lives of others? Or should scientists come to terms with those fears and ask if the resulting *good* outweighs the possible *bad*? It is the same question exploring minds have faced for centuries.

Chapter 2

The Charismatic Stem Cell

*W*hat is it about these tiny chambers that are so intriguing? What do they look like? Where does one find them? How are they already influencing everyday life? Before we address the compelling side of stem cell medicine, it is helpful to know what a stem cell is – and what it isn't. Very succinctly, we define stem cells.

What is a Stem Cell?

Not every cell in a person's body is a stem cell, but *every* body has stem cells. Stem cells have three special qualities. They can divide indefinitely. They can turn into other types of cells. They can repair themselves and therefore, potentially repair the body. Stem cells are located in all areas of the body including the blood, organs, and tissue — however, some of these areas are richer with stem cells than others.

Are Humans the Only Species to Have Stem Cells?

Stem cells originate from three sources: you (these are called autologous cells); from another person (called allogeneic cells); and from non-human sources such as a plant or an animal (called xenogeneic cells).

Are there Different Kinds of Human Stem Cells?

Nature creates two different kinds of stem cells: embryonic and adult stem cells.

What are *Embryonic* Stem Cells?

In simplistic terms, they are stem cells that exist prior to birth. As schoolchildren we are taught that, when male sperm fertilizes a female egg, an embryo is formed. In truth, it isn't quite this simple or immediate. It will take a week after fertilization for pre-embryonic development to occur. At day three, called cleavage, only 16 cells exist, At four or five days, called the blastocyst, 50 to 150 cells have formed.

The blastocyst is an exciting stage of cell development. This is where it becomes possible to distinguish conventional cells from stem cells. Conventional cells have a specific makeup that determines exactly what type of cell each will be. For instance, a conventional blood cell will only become a blood cell; a conventional brain cell can only become a brain cell; and this is the way it is with all non-stem cells found throughout the body. Stem cells, however, have the potential to be *pluripotent*. This means that it is possible to redirect stem cells so that they become other kinds of cells more useful to the body.

At four or five days of age, a blastocyst is not a fully formed embryo. That won't happen until about 10 days later.

What are *Adult* Stem Cells?

It follows that if embryonic stem cells are those existing prior to birth, then adult stem cells are those existing *after* birth. Their primary functions are to maintain a steady habitat so that cells can function as they should and to replace cells that die because of injury or disease.

What is the Physical Makeup of a Stem Cell?

Stem cells range in consistency and size. Some are very rigid and others are spongy. Biomedical engineers at Brown University found that they could predict whether the cells would become bone, cartilage, or fat, based on their consistency and size. By viewing stem cells in petri dishes, they discovered that the rigid cells were generally smaller and transformed into bone. The spongiest cells were the largest and became fat tissue, while the stickiest cells grew into cartilage.

To put stem cell size into perspective, it helps to visualize everyday objects. The average stem cell is about 11 microns in size; a micron being a linear measurement equal to one-millionth of a meter. By comparison, a grain of sand is about 100 microns — nearly 10 times bigger than a stem cell. A strand of hair is about 40 to 50 microns in diameter and therefore about 4 times bigger than a stem cell. However in the environment of a petri dish, stem cells do outrank other matter in size: the smaller red blood cell is only about 6-10 microns; bacteria are smaller still at about 5 microns; and a virus is a very diminutive .05 of a micron.

Where Does One Find Stem Cells?

Adult stem cells are rare, yet they exist everywhere in the body. They are more abundant in bone marrow, blood, skin, and teeth. The mandibular third molar is rich with stem cells, enough so that it could eventually supply a minimum of 29 different end organs. To better understand how rare stem cells are: each milliliter of bone marrow contains approximately six million cells (6,000,000); however, no more than sixty thousand (60,000) of them are stem cells. (Less than 1%). Even rarer, one out of one-hundred-thousand (100,000) cells in the blood stream is a stem cell.

How Are Adult Stem Cells Extracted from the Body?

Generally they are removed surgically. Stem cells in the heart and brain are removed by biopsy, as are stem cells in the skin. Stem cells in the ovaries exist in the eggs, which can be gently suctioned out, non-surgically. Stem cells in bone marrow are removed either by biopsy (which extracts small samples of bone plus the fluid and cells of the marrow) or through aspiration which extracts only the marrow fluid and cells.

Do Adult Stem Cells Exist in Fat?

Adult stem cells are plentiful in fat and once these stem cells are transformed, they are showing great promise in their ability to benefit the body. In terms of availability, each gram of fat contains about two million cells and approximately 10% of these are stem cells — far more than the number of stem cells found in bone marrow! To extract human stem cells, doctors used the same liposuction procedures that have become accepted in cosmetic plastic surgery, only in modified proportions.

Are Doctors Transferring Harvested Fat Stem Cells to Other Areas of the Body?

Yes, research in fat transfer has actually progressed beyond the fat harvesting stage to the point where doctors are re-injecting the stem cell-rich fat into damaged areas of the body and studying the results. At UCLA, scientists used fat tissue to grow bone. This bone formed faster and was of a higher quality than bone cultivated through traditional methods. The procedure may one day eliminate painful bone grafts. It has the potential to be especially useful when a patient doesn't have good quality bone to graft or when time is a critical.

Where Do Doctors Find Risk Takers Willing to Subject their Bodies to New Stem Cell Therapies?

Their existing patients often have good reasons to take risks — many times because they have run out of other options. Celebrity sports figures (who are accustomed to taking risks on and off the playing field) are also often willing to try something new because, once they are injured, their multi-million dollar careers are in jeopardy and players know they must return to the team quickly or forfeit the season. An Australian Football League defender, Clint Bartram, underwent a low-risk experimental procedure in the summer of 2012. Doctors harvested fat stem cells and injected them into his degenerative knee. With time, the physicians hoped his knee would regenerate healthy cartilage tissue. NFL football players Peyton Manning and Terrell Owens also pioneered stem cell therapies, traveling outside the United States for treatments not yet approved by the Food and Drug Administration (FDA). Manning, plagued by neck injury, sought treatment in Europe, while Owens turned to doctors in Korea to enhance the tendons in his surgically repaired ACL (knee).

Where Do Research Stem Cells Come From?

When a woman is trying to have a child through in vitro fertilization, she undergoes clinical processes that encourage her body to produce multiple eggs, yet not all of these eggs are fertilized or implanted. She may decide to bank some of the unused eggs, freezing and storing them for future use when she wants to have another child. If she chooses not to become pregnant again, the eggs are discarded. These clinically processed eggs contain useable stem cells. When discarded, they are given to research facilities to create new stem cell lines.

Stem Cells, like all other cells, contain the DNA roadmap to a person's individual make up, however, they are elite cells, capable of far more than ordinary cells. From birth through adulthood, stem cells are worth exploring, saving, and protecting.

If I were Pregnant or going to Become Pregnant, what would I Want to Do Immediately to Help my Baby have a Healthier Start in Life?

Healthy babies come from healthy parents. Before you plan to get pregnant, make sure both parties have healthy lifestyles. This means eating nutritiously and consuming the appropriate number of calories for your body. Sleep is one of life's natural protectors for your body. Honor a regular sleep schedule and aim for approximately 8 hours each night. De-stress as well, to allow the baby growing inside of you to develop without the obstacles created by stress hormones. Moreover, both parents should try to eliminate unhealthy habits, such as smoking, alcohol consumption, and recreational drug use. From this day forward, everything you do has the potential to affect your baby's cells and stem cells.

Can Adult Stem Cells be extracted from a Baby's Umbilical Cord?

The umbilical cord — which is the cord that connects mother and baby in the uterus and supplies nutrients to the baby prior to birth — is detached once the baby is born, allowing the baby to live freely from its mother. After birth, the unattached cord remains a rich source of stem cells and this is one reason umbilical cord blood banks exist — to store the cord's blood and/or stem cells for potential use later in the baby's life. In addition, once a baby is born, the protective sac that surrounds it prior to birth, called the placenta, is naturally expelled from the body and it is also an excellent source for stem cells. (Even menstrual blood contains stem cells.)

What More Would I Want to Know about Stem Cells to Protect my Baby at Birth?

At birth, the mother has the option of saving the umbilical cord at a private banking company, in case the baby acquires a serious or no-hope disease in the future. In the United States, the current procedure is to freeze the whole umbilical cord, thaw it and use a portion of the blood when needed. In some countries (but not the United States), the mother can save both the umbilical cord and placenta. Countries highly advanced in stem cell research are offering still a more sophisticated form of protection. It involves isolating stem cells from the umbilical cord lining and placenta, and banking these stem cells for future use. This procedure is not available in the United States at this time.

Should I Make Use of the Banking Option?

Absolutely, you should save as much as your doctor and your country will allow. Science is taking huge steps in eliminating disease. Researchers with a global reach now believe that it is better to save the stem cells directly because they are more advantageous than saving the umbilical cord blood alone and they offer much more potential for the future. Many researchers in the United States believe that the day this country allows you to save the baby's isolated stem cells, *you simply must!*

Why?

After 20 years, your baby's umbilical cord will be discarded because there is no proof as to whether or not it is safe to use after so much time has elapsed. However, it is not until later in life that most serious diseases becomes apparent — and that's when a person could really use a boost from his or her early, undamaged, stem cells.

In some countries, doctors already isolate these stem cells for indefinite use — far beyond 20 years. It works like this. A cell is isolated and allowed to divide up to four times, creating four generations of this cell. At each division (or generation), the stem cell is frozen to stop it from dividing further and it is transferred to a vial. Should the baby's stem cells ever be needed to fight disease, doctors would turn to the fourth generation first, and if need be, the third and then the second. If the first cell was needed, it would be allowed to divide first, thereby creating an infinite supply of a person's own early stem cells.

How Can We Be Certain the Stem Cells Saved Belong to my Baby?

Stem cells, DNA, and gene-mapping go hand in hand. Your baby's stem cells contain his DNA and it is as individual to him as his fingerprints. Many decades later, gene-mapping can still identify the DNA make up of a stem cell and confirm whether or not it belongs to your child.

Do our Body's Stem Cells Change as We Grow Older?

As we age, stem cells retain the ability to divide indefinitely. They also continue to repair and grow into other types of cells. However, the number of stem cells that the body produces lessens as we get older. It will take the stem cells of a 50 year-old person approximately 61 hours to double in number, but only about 43 hours to do the same in a healthy 20 year-old. The quality of the stem cells is also affected by aging. Stem cells acquired later in life may not be as vibrant or as healthy as they were when we were younger.

Can a Person's Stem Cells be Transferred Successfully to Another Family Member to Help Save their Life?

Before stem cells are injected into someone else's body, both donor and receiver undergo complex testing in much the same way organ transplant donors and recipients do, to be sure their organs are a match with little cause for rejection. There are many factors that determine a good match, including blood type and the presence of similar antibodies.

The chances are one in four that you would be a direct match for another family member. If you both have the diseased gene, your stem cells will transfer the gene to them as well. In that case, your stem cells would not be of value. Before any stem cells could be transferred, both donor and recipient would undergo essential testing to determine if the transplant should take place.

Could Acquiring Younger Stem Cells Make an Older Person Younger?

Researchers *are* looking for the fountain of youth in stem cells! They hope to one day implant younger cells into receptive older bodies for both health and beauty benefits. The experimentation currently requires more development; however, it has been proven that when an older stem cell is surrounded with younger stem cells in a petri dish, the older stem cell begins to act younger. Conversely, when a younger stem cell is introduced to older stem cells, the younger stem cells act more mature. (*See Aging in the Disease Section.*) How ironic that this practice also happens socially with people!

Once Stem Cells are Introduced in a Body, Can they be Rejected?

When blood or blood products are absent, there is little chance of rejection. This is why fat and skin are excellent sources of stem cells. Once the stem cells are extracted and purified, there are no blood products remaining. The chances of rejection are very small to nil, especially when the cells are from one's own body.

Are Some Stem Cells Better to Transplant than Others?

Doctors select stem cells that are not too old and not too young. They want to know that the cells they select are destined to become the kind of cells needed — that is, that they have begun to differentiate in a given direction. If the stem cells are to be used to repair the brain they must be identifiable as neural stem cells; if needed to repair the heart, they must be differentiating as heart muscle cells. Doctors can also coax cells to grow in a given direction. By adding the right nutrients to the stem cells as they grow in a petri dish, or by changing their genetic makeup, doctors can create cells that are more ideal for a transplant.

If Stem Cells can become Other Types of cells, can they turn into Cancer Cells?

Yes, but the possibility of getting cancer from a stem cell transplant is remote unless the person providing the stem cells already has cancer or is in the process of developing it. This is an important reason donors are closely evaluated before becoming a patient match.

Can a Person get a Benign Tumor from a Stem Cell Transplant?

Teratomas multiply randomly and aggressively like cancer, but they are not malignant cancer; they are benign tumors. Teratomas form when very young embryonic stem cells differentiate in the wrong direction and continue growing down the wrong path. They are masses of cells disorganized in their growth, sometimes containing such wayward origins as teeth or hair. Because teratomas are not stem cells, they would not even be considered for a stem cell transplant.

Does Cancer have Stem Cells?

This can be confusing. Cancer cells are not stem cells by default because they lack one of the three basic functions that define a stem cell. True, they can reproduce indefinitely and they can differentiate into other kinds of cells, but they cannot repair themselves or the body. But cancer does have stem cells *within* it. Think of these stem cells as mother cells. A mother cell can continue to reproduce indefinitely, it can mutate or differentiate, and although it doesn't repair the host body (the person with cancer), it can suck up the nutrition the host needs to repair its own corrupt cells so that they survive.

In Science Fiction, Cancer Cells are used as Weapons. Can a Stem Cell be turned into a Cancer Cell and therefore a Weapon?

There is not enough information known about stem cells now to take a stem cell and deliberately turn it into a cancer cell. Even though an undifferentiated stem cell can become other kinds of stem cells, scientists still can't take a stem cell and turn it into anything they want it to be.

Chapter 3

Giving Stem Cells their Due

*S*tem cells are thought to have been identified as early as the mid-1800s, when German scientists presumed their existence after studying developing embryos and microscopic views of bone marrow. It wasn't until after World War II, however, that the modern day scientific community acquired a passionate interest in stem cell research — for the sake of humanity.

What Have We Learned from Hiroshima and Nagasaki?

An estimated 225,000 people lost their lives in the combined bombings of Hiroshima and Nagasaki (Japan), nearly 20% of them in prolonged deaths due to radiation poisoning. Radiation damages the body in a systemized order: first it kills white blood cells, then it affects the gastro-intestinal track, and then — with higher dosages as a result of longer radiation exposure (or) the exposure that would come from being located closest to the bombed site — it affects the neurological system.

After the bombings, some individuals died immediately because they could no longer regenerate adequate white blood cells to fight infection, nor did they have enough platelets to allow their blood to clot properly. Those who lived but who experienced higher doses of radiation saw damage to their intestinal tracks. Many of those who lived for long periods after the bombings experienced blood cancers and leukemia.

17

Could Stem Cells Have Helped this Situation?

Horrific as they were, the bombings allowed researchers to make important discoveries about radiation and its effects on the body. It would take until the year 1956 to show that bone marrow injected with new stem cells could rejuvenate human blood-forming systems. This was the beginning of modern-day bone marrow transplants. *(See 'What is a bone marrow transplant?')*

Over the next five years, stem cell research continued — progressing in painstakingly small steps, most often at the expense of the mouse population. In fact, mice were (and still are) the unsung heroes of stem cell research since very little research has been done on humans that hasn't first been perfected on mice. By 1961 Canadian researchers understood the properties of transplantable stem cells in the bone marrow of mice. They also learned how to establish *colonies* of stem cells (in mice) and created a methodology for counting them. This was an important discovery, one that made all other stem cell research possible.

What Other Countries were Involved in Early Stem Cell Research?

In 1978, researchers in the United States recognized transplantable stem cells in human cord blood. Beginning in 1982, the United Kingdom and the United States developed methodology to genetically modify embryonic stem cells. By 1994, Taiwanese doctors were successful in treating patients with damaged corneas, using cornea stem cells. In 2006, researchers in Japan reprogrammed adult mouse skin cells, creating induced pluripotent stem cells (iPS) with characteristics similar to embryonic stem cells.

And Now?

Stem cell research has exploded worldwide. One estimate indicates that there may be as many as 200,000 stem cell studies currently taking place, in countries that are determined to be twenty-first century science leaders. Using gene mapping, DNA research, and stem cell research,

these researchers are intent on finding the cure for no-hope diseases —
and solutions that will make life better.

How do Researchers Classify Stem Cells?

There are two distinct classifications of stem cells, based on the type of cell each has the potential to become. There are Hematopoietic stem cells and Mesenchymal stem cells.

What are Hematopoietic Stem Cells?

Hematopoietic means *blood* and so it follows that these stem cells are crucial to the body's blood supply. The average person needs an incredible one-hundred-billion new blood cells every day to carry oxygen to the tissues and to fight infection. Some of these blood cells don't live long so they must be replaced constantly. Without Hematopoietic stem cells overseeing the production, new blood cells could not form. Hematopoietic stem cells are located in close proximity to the body's blood cells, making it possible for researchers to coax them into blood vessel cells and the cells of blood products. Additionally, these stem cells transform into cells of the skin and nervous system as well.

What are Mesenchymal Stem Cells?

Mesenchymal stem cells serve as infection-fighters in the body and they are also known to have the properties associated with immunity. This means they work to keep the body free from disease. Mesenchymal stem cells are located at the entrance and exit of the bone marrow cavity, making it possible for them to interact easily with other cells as they enter the cavity. Like Hematopoietic stem cells, Mesenchymal stem cells are capable of becoming blood vessel cells and cells of the nervous system, but they can also transform into organs, fat cells, connective tissues, muscle, bone, and blood. In the world of stem cell research, this transformation is known as differentiation.

Do Hematopoietic and Mesenchymal Stem Cells Co-exist?

Generally Hematopoietic stem cells and Mesenchymal stem cells are found together in the body as a mixed group of cells; it is the proportion of each that makes every body part unique. For instance, bone is made up of predominately mesenchymal stem cells, but it also has hematopoietic stem cells in its makeup. No matter where in the body a stem cell originates, it functions like its predominate cells.

How Can Scientists tell if a Stem Cell is Hematopoietic or Mesenchymal?

Every cell type has a certain combination of receptors on its surface that differentiates it from other kinds of cells. When the cells are stained, the receptors are revealed and they can be identified. The receptors are called markers. Markers are named using a combination of the prefix *CD* followed by numbers. When stained, Hematopoietic stem cells reveal the CD45 and CD34 markers. Mesenchymal stem cells reveal markers CD44, CD73, CD90, and CD 105 when stained.

CD is an abbreviation for Cluster of Differentiation. The number following CD is a universal code given to a particular molecule found on the surface of a cell. By the year 2009, more than 350 unique surface molecules were identified. This system allows the scientific community to refer to stem cells using one universal language.

Do Scientists favor using Hematopoietic or Mesenchymal Stem Cells in their Studies?

Given that they have a choice — based on the type of experiments they are conducting — researchers often favor Mesenchymal stem cells. They are bigger in size and that makes them easier to work with. There are also many more of them in the body, so they are easier to access. Bone marrow (consisting predominately of Hematopoietic stem cells) is more limited in what can be derived from it. The larger cells in fat (Mesenchymal stem cells) make it more ideal for research.

What is a Unipotent Stem Cell?

Unipotent stem cells can only be coaxed (altered) into one specific type of stem cell.

What are Multipotent Stem Cells?

Multi means more than one. Multipotent stem cells can be coaxed into more than one kind of cell. Multipotent stem cells are more limited in their possibilities than pluripotent stem cells.

What are Pluripotent Stem Cells?

These stem cells can become almost any kind of stem cell.

What are Induced Pluripotent Stem Cells (iPS)?

These are the now famous embryonic-like stem cells that resulted from the research of Nobel Prize recipient Shinya Yamanaka. Researchers use adult stem cells, generally from skin, and return them to their near-embryonic stage without ever touching an embryo.

Do Researchers Study Stem Cells Solely for the Purpose of Preventing Disease?

Preventing disease is enormously important. However, some study stem cells to better understand human development and our species. Regardless of religious indoctrination or political affirmation, *all* people benefit when we know more about what makes us human. Studying embryonic stem cells gives researchers the unique advantage of scrutinizing important functions of the human body — especially the brain — without invasive manipulation of the body itself.

Do Researchers Clone Diseased Cells?

Yes, when a diseased cell is cloned, researchers can watch how the new cell develops. They look for the exact moment disease is apparent. In evaluating that moment, it is possible to get to the heart of the illness and its cause — and that gives researchers the best chance of curing it.

Why Did a Controversy Erupt over the Cloning (also called nuclear transfer) of Embryonic Stem Cells?

The philosophies of the world's religions vary but some religions, including Catholicism and the more fundamentalist Christian faiths, refuse to sanction the practice of embryonic stem cell transfer because they believe that life begins at the moment of conception — the moment the sperm and egg combine, which is also known as fertilization.

Not all religions and cultures, nor science, agree with this definition. Jewish theology honors the developing fetus, but believes that it will take 45 days for the embryo to achieve personhood. In Islamic religion, life begins in the fourth month of pregnancy. The exact moment of personhood has been debated philosophically and scientifically for centuries. Some believe life begins at the first heartbeat, others at the first appearance of brain waves or when the central nervous system in a fetus is mature. Still others believe life stirs at the quickening when the fetus begins to move. There are those who subscribe to the idea that until a fetus is capable of feeling pain, or until it can survive outside of the womb, it is not a living human being. With so many options, the answer remains simple for some. Life begins at the moment of birth.

Why Is the Defining Moment of Life so Important?

During embryonic stem cell transfer, the outer layer of the pre-embryonic blastocyst is destroyed. Those adhering to the narrowest definition of life equate the death of this cell with the death of a fully formed fetus.

It should be noted here that even nature prohibits many pre-embryonic blastocysts from developing further. This early in a pregnancy, a spontaneous miscarriage can happen without a woman even knowing she is pregnant. In addition, while a religion or culture may subscribe to a particular doctrine, many within their ranks actually practice a variation of the moral code. For example, the Catholic Church does not sanction the use of birth control, yet within the ranks of its most faithful, there are those committed to its use. Perhaps most understandable, fundamentally-raised parents of congenitally ill children do not necessarily favor religious doctrine over the science of stem cells when the goal is to keep their severely ill children alive!

How Do These Parents Justify the Seemingly Conflicting Views?

Some simply accept that God sent the stem cells. Scientifically, it sometimes comes down to this: an embryo cannot grow to become a living child without first being nourished and sustained. Therefore, the embryo becomes the *possibility* of life, but not life itself. Likewise, the embryo holds the *possibility* of becoming a stem cell and with it, the *possibility* for curing illness. Viewed this way, a stem cell has options. It can create a new life or it can save one.

During the George W. Bush presidency (2001-2009), we heard much about stem cell lines.

What Are Stem Cell Lines?

A stem cell line is a group of related cells that are constantly dividing. They are derived from a single stem cell.

What are the Often-Referenced 60 *Embryonic Stem Cell Lines*?

Former United States President George Bush opposed stem cell research derived from human embryos, choosing instead to believe the most conservative definition of life: that it begins at conception. Based on his personal beliefs and with the support of his conservative political base, he banned the use of Federal funds for research on human embryonic stem cells.

Excluded from this ban were 60 privately funded stem cell lines that already existed. In a speech before the American public, Bush concluded that the life-and-death decision pertaining to these stem cells had already been made. In his mind, these embryos had already been destroyed. Therefore, it was in the public's best interest to continue using them for exploration purposes so that some good might come from their existence.

In 2009, newly-elected President Barack Obama repealed the ban.

Why Weren't Researchers Content to Experiment on 60 Lines?

While it is true that stem cells can reproduce indefinitely, it is also true that each new generation of cells ages and changes. Stem cells are constantly trying to do what stem cells naturally do — differentiate into the type of cell each wants to be. As the 60 lines continued to grow, the cells also experience deterioration. To be medically useful, researchers needed access to the highest quality stem cells possible. In short, they needed fresh lines.

Where Did these Lines Originate and Did that Create Problems?

The stem cell lines were derived from embryos that had been donated to researchers by infertility clinics (as most research stem cells are). The purpose of infertility clinics is to help women get pregnant when they are having trouble conceiving. To produce these embryos, the clinics pump a woman's body full of hormones to help her body prepare for conception. This created another reason for researchers to request other lines. Due to the manipulations prior to the creation of the original 60 lines, they were not a true representation of nature — or the population as a whole. They existed with their own bias, creating caveats for widespread study.

Furthermore, a woman desiring to have a baby also tends to be younger in age, harboring the cells and potential diseases that are reflective of her age. Researchers wanted additional stem cell lines donated by people of all ages, especially seniors, because that's when many serious diseases like Parkinson's and heart damage become apparent.

How Many Stem Cell Lines Exist Now?

There were more than 180 lines listed in the National Human Embryonic Stem Cell Registry near the end of 2012. The registry is overseen by the NIH — the National Institute of Health — and covers stem cell lines available to researchers from around the world.

Who is Leading the Way in the Registration of Stem Cell Lines?

England has numerous lines registered but the bulk of lines in the registry originate in the United States. Many are established by prominent medical schools such as Harvard University, The University of Michigan, The Rockefeller University, and New York University School of Medicine. Other lines originate at well-known medical facilities such as The Children's Hospital Corporation and Cedars-Sinai Medical Center. Still others are registered to innovative medical corporations including GENEA, BioTime, Inc., and Reprogenetics, LLC.

What is Important About these Stem Cell Lines?

Some of the lines will be used as a control group as they appear to be disease-free. They may also be used for the study of healthy cells. Many of the other stem cell lines have been preserved so that researchers may explore a particular disease. The lines are as diversified as the researchers who study them. For instance, there is a stem cell line that carries a genetic mutation found in Huntington's Disease, a hereditary disease that can eventually make a person unable to talk and walk. There is also a line that carries a genetic mutation for hemophilia, a hereditary condition that prohibits blood clotting. One line was preserved to study heart muscles that grow rigid and weaken in young athletes who die suddenly and unexpectedly.

In order to obtain these stem cell lines, patients with a specific disease have donated their stem cells. The cells are then differentiated into many types of cells — heart, liver, tissue, blood, etc.

Keep in mind that other countries and other companies are developing stem cell lines as well. The NIH registry lists only stem cell lines approved for Federal funding in the United States.

Who Has Been a Prominent Funder of Stem Cell Research?

In the U.S., the NIH is seen as the leader in research funding; however, some calculations indicate the California Institute for Regenerative Medicine (CIRM) has surpassed NIH when all grants are considered beginning as far back as 2007. CIRM was created as a direct result of California's Proposition 71, a 2004 referendum passed by voters specifically to foster stem cell research during the period of declining research in the Bush presidency. CIRM was designated as the overseer and distributer of $3 billion in state funding that was to be spread over a 10 year period.

What has CIRM funded?

In many cases, it has awarded grants for infrastructure and training, including new lab space and faculty for research. It has also funded specific studies.

Has CIRM Influenced the Direction of Research Based on its Grant Approvals?

During its first year of grants (2007), financial support was given unilaterally to embryonic stem cell research. This was the early days of research when embryonic stem cells seemed to hold the greatest potential for success. By 2008, CIRM was already funding research in adult pluripotent stem cells. The bulk of funding continued to center on embryonic stem cells, however.

By 2009, CIRM's focus evolved from purely studying the cells to putting discoveries into clinical application. Grants to develop Translational Medicine (See *Translational Medicine*) studies began to appear. The goal was to bring clinical trials and therapies to doctors in the shortest period safely possible. In this period, more emphasis was placed on adult and pluripotent stem cell funding. The trend continued into 2012.

While CIRM funding has influenced the path of research, specifically by supporting the early years of embryonic stem cell study, it has also been responsible for the development of more publicly accepted research, which will ultimately bring new solutions to patients much quicker.

Chapter 4

Cloning and Stem Cells

*W*e are witnessing a world that looks much different than the one our parents knew ...

Are *Coaxing* Stem Cells and Genetic Engineering — One and the Same?

No, but the development of each has influenced the other and both sciences have made tremendous advancements over the last two decades.

What is the Difference, then, between Altering (Coaxing) a Stem Cell and Conducting Genetic Engineering?

In the right environment (such as in a petri dish prepared with the proper nutrients), stem cells can be coaxed into different kinds of cells in order to alter their purpose. The type of cell that they become varies (i.e. heart, bone, liver, blood, etc.), but the DNA found in the stem cell remains the same. Typically, the new purpose of the stem cell is to function in an area near the site where the original cell was taken, for example, a stem cell from the aorta might be coaxed into becoming tissue for one of the heart chambers. DNA can be taken out of a stem cell and later put back in, however, unless it is genetically engineered, that DNA is not altered.

Genetic engineering is the direct manipulation of the genome (genes). In other words, adding DNA that is taken from another person's cells changes the DNA code of the original cell so it becomes genetically different.

Are Stem Cell Alteration and Cloning the Same?

No, but researchers may use a combination of both to further their efforts. In addition, they might also introduce genetic engineering, utilizing all three or any combination of the three.

Then what is Cloning?

Cloning is the creation of an exact copy of a cell (or an entity).

Identical twins are a natural clone in the human population. Although they are not really 100% identical, they are nearly so. Some plants and bacteria reproduce asexually and these are considered natural clones as well.

Researchers clone cells so that they have a common base to work from. For instance, if two identically-cloned cells are subjected to different treatments and the results are different, researches know it was the treatment that affected the change — and not the cell itself.

Dolly, the first fully-cloned mammal, was an adult ewe cloned from another ewe using her mammillary stem cells.

How did Dolly Come to Be?

Scottish embryologist Ian Wilmut had a research conundrum that he was trying to resolve. As a genetic engineer, he was challenged to develop hybrid sheep that could produce milk enhanced with antibiotics and proteins. The milk, once purified, would be beneficial for people with Cystic Fibrosis and other lung diseases.

Wilmut first created a ewe named Tracy — only one of 1,000 embryos to survive the genetically engineered feat of combining egg and sperm with the AAT gene. (The AAT gene's function is to create proteins that hinder lung tissue deterioration.) In the truest sense, Tracy was not a clone; she was a *chimera* — the name given to organisms with two or more genetically-different (DNA) tissues.

The hybrid-Tracy produced 35 times the amount of AAT typically found in ewes and for this reason Wilmut's experiment was a success. However, because only one embryo in the experiment was capable of accepting the AAT gene, the process needed to be perfected before it could supply the human population with enough enriched milk to benefit anyone's breathing difficulties. Wilmut reasoned the best way to move forward was to clone embryos capable of accepting the AAT gene.

So How did Wilmut Clone a Sheep?

The colossal accomplishment occurred once Ian Wilmut perceived old knowledge in a new way and linked it together with the insight of others who had been focusing on smaller pieces of the creation puzzle. Wilmut began with the earlier works of Sir John Gurdon of England, who cloned the first tadpole in the 1960s by removing the nucleus of a cell and replacing it with another genetically (DNA) altered cell. This is called nuclear transfer or somatic cell nuclear transfer.

Do you see how ideas travel through both time and the scientific community? This is the same John Gurdon who was honored in 2012 with *the Nobel Prize in Physiology or Medicine*, the very same researcher who also influenced Yamanaka's work in the development of the induced pluripotent stem cell (iPS).

Like Gurdon and his tadpoles, Wilmut exchanged the nucleus of a sheep's cell with an embryonic stem cell – providing the cell with the ability to differentiate into other kinds of cells. Though it sounds simple, it would not be an easy leap from the cloning of frogs to the cloning of a mammal. Cloning a mammal is much more complex.

The discoveries of other brilliant minds also made important contributions that helped to shape Dolly. From Steen Willadsen, Wilmut learned more about the properties of embryonic stem cells; from Leroy

Stevens, he learned that tissue could contain various types of cells — muscle, bone, skin, teeth and others. Gail Martin and Martin Evans proved that different cell types began as undifferentiated cells; and they discovered how to grow (mouse) embryos in a petri dish using a special combination of nutrients, cells, and nurturing sera — a practice that would foreshadow Wilmut's own cultivations. Keith Campbell discovered the significance of synchronizing the cycles of donor and recipient cells. Others too, contributed information large and small.

All told, it took the scientific community 30 years of trial and error to advance from the cloning of tadpoles to the cloning of a sheep. While there have been attempts in the cloning of a human, none have proven successful or legitimate. It must be noted that should human cloning ever be accomplished, the process will be much more demanding than the one Ian Wilmut faced when cloning a sheep.

What was Dolly's Ultimate Impact on the Science of Stem Cells?

In developing the ewe, Ian Wilmut not only created the first cloned mammal, but he also identified two important trails for future scientists to pursue. Wilmut proved that adult stem cells could be reprogrammed. He also laid the foundation to explore *human* embryonic stem cells with all their incredible possibilities.

Did the Scientific Community Pause Then to Examine the Ethics of Cloning a Human Being?

Definitely. In scientific labs around the world researchers asked the ultimate question: was it morally ethical to clone a human being? Most concluded that cloning for reproductive purposes was unethical.

What is Reproductive Cloning?

The purpose of human reproductive cloning is to bring a new, genetically identical person to life, capable of living and breathing as a complete, self-sustaining Individual. It is believed by most scientists —

and the general public alike — that this practice speaks of human vanity and/or of 'playing God'.

However, most in the scientific community do believe that therapeutic cloning has the potential to ease human suffering — and it is in that spirit that the research advances.

What is Therapeutic Cloning?

Therapeutic cloning exists to better mankind. It does not clone entire human beings. It clones a limited quantity of specific cells. The goal of therapeutic cloning is to find cures for diseases. Beyond this, researchers envision a day when they will grow new tissue and organs, preferably from a patient's own body, to replace damaged, missing, and diseased body parts.

But Can't Patients Opt for a Donor Transplant Instead?

Each month about 4,100 people are added to the United States' transplant waiting list. During 2012, more than 105,000 patients were anxiously waiting for that gift that would save their lives. In the United States where individuals and families *do* generously donate organs, approximately 77 patients receive new organs daily. Still, 18 others die because of limited availabilities. Sadly, there aren't enough transplantable organs for all the people who need them.

When Stem Cells are Cloned, Can They Actually Be Used in Medical Practice?

The FDA must approve all medical trials and procedures in the United States before they can be implemented in patient use. Currently only *minimally manipulated* procedures have been approved. Furthermore, researchers are forbidden to bank or culture stem cells for complex procedures here.

Where Do Other Countries Stand in their Stem Cell Capabilities?

China's government has strongly supported the study of regenerative medicine, which includes not only stem cell research but gene therapy and tissue engineering as well. It has made healthcare research a priority since the year 2000 and has become one of the five largest publishers of peer-reviewed scientific papers globally, surpassed only by the United Kingdom, Japan, Germany, and the United States. Although American researchers out-publish their Chinese counterparts, China's scientists are delivering stem cell applications more quickly.

How can China do this?

During the George W. Bush stem cell prohibition, the Chinese government saw its opportunity to become a world leader in healthcare. It actively recruited and developed researchers to study stem cells and, just as importantly, it provided adequate long-term funding for the program. (One only needs to look at China's competitive Olympic sports teams to understand the expectations it has for its people and the commitment it is willing to make to get the job done.) China was also able to place fewer restraints on its researchers, in part, because the Chinese religion does not bestow personhood on an embryo. Additionally, China made it a priority to bring new stem cell therapies to fruition quickly.

Didn't that Result in Inferior Medical Practices?

Prior to 2009, dual research tracks existed. Top-quality regenerative medicine research was produced by China's academic institutions, national research centers, and a few small firms, just as it has been in the United States. Quality issues developed because the limited governmental regulations also allowed some firms, and even a number of hospitals, to market their therapies without scientific evidence to back them up. Market them they did! These unproven sources created a tourist industry targeting vulnerable patients around the world who were suffering from no-hope diseases, promising treatment for everything from Parkinson's, to multiple sclerosis, to diabetes, and cerebral palsy.

Since then, the Ministry of Health in China has adopted new rules which require stem cell centers to provide safety and efficiency evidence for their protocols; however, full compliance has not been achieved. Medical tourists are warned to beware — and to seek out China's top-quality practitioners, just as you would here at home.

Are there Smaller Countries Surpassing the U.S. in Stem Cell Applications?

Doctors extract stem cells from the peripheral blood in one arm of a Leukemia patient, by stimulate, concentrate and activate the white blood cells and then re-inject the stem cells into the patient's other arm. This procedure is reminiscent of one used in dialysis treatment in the United States. Currently, this stem cell protocol has only been approved by the FDA for a very limited number of conditions in the United States, including Leukemia. However, in other countries in South America, this procedure has been used for the treatment of many more conditions besides Leukemia with promising results.

If the United States is going to become a leader in stem cell medicine, researchers in conjunction with the FDA must work quickly to catch up.

Chapter 5

The Importance of Advocates

*P*erhaps no one is more receptive to therapeutic cloning than parents whose children are inflicted with debilitating no-hope diseases, followed closely by adults who have been touched by serious disease themselves. For them, it isn't necessary to reconcile their beliefs in science, religion, and politics; their only desire is to save a life.

Even the most devout religious or anti-political practitioner has been known to have a change of heart about stem cells when faced with a personal — and unbearable — medical catastrophe. When that someone happens to be a public figure, his or her grief can help others understand a previously unimaginable view. Grief can forge bonds between the most unlikely candidates; on a more practical note, it can also generate much needed funding. By sharing their intensely private and personal stories, public persons have the ability to rally new hope for others afflicted by the same disease.

How Did First Lady Nancy Reagan Become a Believer?

Former First Lady Nancy Reagan had an abrupt change of heart once she became her husband's first line of defense against Alzheimer's disease. Prior to his diagnosis, both she and President Ronald Reagan had been unwavering anti-abortionists whose pro-life viewpoints spilled over into their stance against embryonic stem cell research. They considered this developing new science an affront against life. By 1988 the then-President had banned Federal funding for research pertaining to the transplant of embryos. Without funding, stem cell study came to a halt in the United States. By 2004, Ronald Reagan had been battling Alzheimer's for ten years and his memory was no longer functional. He was unable to recall his White House experiences as well as those he lovingly shared with his family.

Did She Voice her Support?

In April 2004, knowing that then-President George W. Bush and his administration were debating whether to halt embryonic stem cell research in the United States, Mrs. Reagan wrote a letter to President Bush in support of stem cell research, acknowledging, "Ronnie struggles in a world unknown to me or the scientists who devote their lives to Alzheimer's research. Because of this, I am determined to do what I can to save others from this pain and anguish."

By May, she had become a vocal advocate for stem cells as well. Speaking publicly at a ceremony before the Juvenile Diabetes Research Foundation she announced, "Science has presented us with a hope called stem cell research, which may provide our scientists with answers that have so long been beyond our grasp. I just don't see how we can turn our backs on this. We have lost so much time already."

She was not the only public face to champion the stem cell cause.

Examine the involvement of actors Michael J. Fox and the late Christopher Reeve and you discover a new respect for the two men who used their celebrity-status to advocate for an ailing population.

What has Michael J. Fox Done for Stem Cell Research?

When science cures the disease, every Parkinson's patient will owe Michael J. Fox a debt of gratitude. He won't have helped to achieve the cure without the input of many others, but he is hugely responsible for mobilizing researchers and the critical resources they need. When researchers needed governmental support, or money, or clinical trials, or participants for those trials, Fox found them through the Foundation he created that bears his name.

Realistically, Michael J. Fox wants a cure for Parkinson's, regardless of whether it's through the use of stem cells or not. He has testified before United States legislators concerning the need for innovative exploration. Since its founding in 2000, the Michael J. Fox Foundation has awarded more than $313 million to Parkinson's research, $56 million in 2012 alone. These grants nurture promising drugs as well as genetic engineering — and stem cell discovery remains an important part of the mix. Fox's legendary support of stem cells has rippled through the philanthropic community, encouraging others to give too.

This year the (New York) Empire State Stem Cell Board recommended funding in the amount of $14.9 million to be awarded to the Memorial Sloan-Kettering Cancer Center for stem cell research, directed toward the study of Parkinson's. Specifically, the study seeks to engineer dopamine-producing cells capable of functioning properly once delivered to the brain. If successful, they will be used to replace a patient's diseased Parkinson's cells. It is the next chapter of a study that began under Fox's earlier financial support.

Has Fox supported embryonic stem cell research?

Yes. In the early days of stem cell therapies, he ardently supported embryonic stem cell therapies, which were thought to hold the key to eradicating Parkinson's. In a CNN Special Report, he told Dr. Sanjay Gupta "patients have the right to insist that Federal funders and industry do anything that's likely to find an answer — to find a cure." He added "to shut off any possible inroad to a cure or breakthrough just seem(s) to make no sense, especially when attached to a political agenda."

But Hasn't He Since Withdrawn his Support for Stem Cell Exploration?

Even into 2013, the Michael J. Fox Foundation website has advocated for the support of researchers, recognizing their need for freedom as they explore embryonic, adult and iPS stem cell possibilities.

Fox has spoken so often and for so long about a cure, that partial statements continue to surface in both traditional and social media. Many times they are presented out of context. Because of this, it is possible to think that Fox has given up on stem cells. In reality, like so many scientific researchers, he has shifted his interest away from embryonic cells to the currently more promising induced pluripotent adult stem cells.

And who is Michael J. Fox?

The Canadian-born actor just might be Parkinson's most famous patient. He is widely known in the United States for his roles in the television sitcoms *Family Ties* and *Spin City*, as well as in the *Back to the Future* movies. After his tremors became severely pronounced, he continued to perform in guest roles on high profile television series. He was diagnosed with Parkinson's at the young age of thirty. With a family in addition to his career success, he believed he still had much living to do and set about doing it. Besides his work at his Foundation, he continues to educate the public about Parkinson's and stem cells through his books: *Lucky Man: A Memoir; A Funny Thing Happened on the Way to the Future: Twists and Turns and Lessons Learned* and *Always Looking Up: The Adventures of an Incurable Optimist*.

What Happened to Christopher Reeve?

The horse that the late Christopher Reeve was riding bucked, trouncing him to the ground, propelling him into the life-altering world of a quadriplegic. For anyone else, this would have been a life-shattering experience, but with the help of a strong wife, his family, and a team of innovative medical researchers, the Superman actor summoned his own heroic powers to redefine himself as a spinal cord injury survivor and advocate.

Why Did He Seek Treatment in Israel?

In 2003, Reeve saw the waning support for stem cell research in the United States, turning to Israel in hopes of finding treatment for his condition. Owing to decades of war conditions, Israel has one of the highest incidents of spinal injury. Traveling there, Reeve found pro-active rehab facilities, excellent medical schools and hospitals, and a praise-worthy infrastructure for research. He toured a facility where children had had stem cell therapies within 14 days of their injuries; he was inspired by the progress in their recoveries.

How did Reeve Further Early Government Backing of Stem Cells?

He had a long history of supporting stem cell research, lobbying for additional Federal funding of embryonic stem cell research, acknowledging that as a country, we shouldn't be in the position of creating embryos just for the purpose of study and manipulation. He found it inexcusable that good embryos were going to waste — referring to the healthy embryos that were literally destroyed by the infertility clinics because they were in excess of their patients' needs.

Reeve lobbied for the Human Cloning Prohibition Act of 2001, which would allow somatic cell nuclear transfer research (the process used to create Dolly), but banned reproductive cloning. His stewardship went far beyond American borders. In 2004 he sent a videotaped message to the United Nations in defense of somatic cell nuclear transfer, which was under threat of extinction by world treaty. Even near death, Reeve urged California voters to support the creation of the California Institute for Regenerative Medicine (CIRM), including funding for stem cell research. Voters approved this proposition less than one month after his death.

Even then-California Governor Arnold Schwarzenegger spoke adamantly in favor of stem cell study saying, "I support stem cell research. I think it is very, very important that the whole nation pulls together on a federal and a state level."

Celebrities lend their presence to the stem cell cause, but it is important to recognize the thousands of hard working not-so-famous advocates who also raise money and create awareness to benefit stem cell research. They man information booths, create websites, and take calls from eager patients-to-be. In the name of non-profit organizations, they sit on boards and committees, raise funds, or educate public audiences. Additionally, many medical professionals donate their time and talents to these organizations in hopes of finding a cure.

Chapter 6

Therapeutic Advances
in Stem Cell Research

nyone who waits anxiously as their loved one undergoes major surgery understands that, inside the hospital walls, time passes awkwardly in warped dimensions. On one hand, some aspects of illness race by much too quickly; yet, on the other, some reveal themselves in an agonizingly slow manner.

Research is like that too, only on a bigger scale. For all the groundbreaking revolutions in stem cell advancement — and there have been many — it is also true that *curing* disease through stem cell therapy is often a long way away. Bringing stem cells from the discovery stage to actual human application is a complex process. Researchers aren't yet able to recreate entire organs, but they are positively impacting cells!

What is Stem Cell Replacement Therapy?

The goal of stem cell replacement therapy is to exchange dysfunctional cells in the body with healthy ones.

Is this Easy?

Not so much. First the new cells have to be genetically engineered to perform all the activities that the healthy cells do, without causing the body to reject them or create inflammation at the cell site. Creating these cells isn't enough. Beyond that, they must be implanted in the body in such a way that the cells will live and grow without uncontrolled growth. Devising the right method for implantation can be a time-consuming hit or miss process.

What are Clinical Trials?

By observing how stem cell therapies work in the human body as opposed to the petri dish, researchers are able to develop solutions with real application value. Some clinical trials are simply observational in nature, while others provide drug or treatment interventions. Clinical trials are conducted in hospitals, universities, and clinics across the country — and are critical to the development of new innovations. Many trials can be documented on the Internet where potential participants can learn about them and then explore the possibility of taking part in the trials with their doctor's advice. There are protections in place to guard against injustices and a potential clinical trial candidate should also inquire about these.

Ironically, 30% of all potential clinical trials (including those with non-stem cell origins) do not come to fruition because enough qualified participants didn't commit to initiate the studies; additionally, 85% of trials finish beyond their expected dates because of recruitment problems. Patients are eager to find cures for their diseases, but before there can be a cure, more patients need to step up and participate in the clinical trials.

What are Double-blind, Randomized Controlled Trials?

There is a psychological phenomenon that can happen once a patient begins treatment. The very act of taking a drug often makes people think they are getting better, whether or not the drug is actually working. This is but one variable in treatment that researchers want to control and so, they create double-blind, randomized controlled trials to address variable issues.

To do this, researchers randomly divide their full group into two smaller groups and instruct all patients to take the drug in identical fashion. In actuality, only one group is given the drug; the other is given a substitute of placebos. The placebos resemble the fully functioning drug, but have no active ingredients that could affect the health of the patients. Only the researcher knows who is taking the actual drug and who isn't. The group taking the placebos becomes the researcher's control group, and all results obtained in the first group are measured against the results of this controlled activity. This process is accepted as objective scientific methodology, and when it is performed correctly, it produces untainted bias.

The major criticism of double-blind trials is that they are time consuming to conduct.

What is Translational Medicine?

Traditionally it has taken ten to twenty years to conduct biomedical research. Translational medicine brings new applications and new pharmaceutical drugs to patients more quickly. Doctors are able to put the knowledge that they learn as they perform a study directly into clinical practice. With translational medicine, there is an emphasis on testing real patients in real-life situations where decisions can be modified to fit the patient and the environment. Translational medicine challenges the traditional approach of randomized double blind trials. It is less costly to conduct and the time saved by shaving years off of a clinical trial means that more people can benefit from the healing outcomes sooner.

Will Recent Stem Cell Research Change the Way Doctors Treat Disease?

By the end of 2012, there were more than 4,252 stem cell studies listed on the United States National Institute of Health's website, www.ClinicalTrials.gov. Some were active and many were even actively recruiting patients. Others had been approved by the FDA, but had not yet begun recruiting participants. Some of these trials had even been terminated, but on a given day in December, there were 1,777 open stem cell studies. The site is continuously updated and people with medical issues are encouraged to use this as a valuable resource.

With so many new studies appearing regularly, a book like this cannot be the latest word on up-to-date stem cell discoveries; that may be better suited to the Internet. To complicate matters, researchers are not always willing to discuss the progress they are making with their trials since research can take many years to complete; furthermore, they are often legally bound to remain silent about their progresses until the funders of their studies are ready to reveal the outcomes. Public acknowledgment frequently happens after their findings have been published by a reputable source or after a new drug or procedure has been patented.

Given those limitations, here are some of the more interesting recent results made public. Remember, stem cell research is still in the infancy stage for many diseases — and testing may not yet have been approved for humans.

Aging: Can Stem Cells Slow the Aging Process?

Aging happens when the body is sluggish in regenerating new tissue and it isn't replaced at the same pace that old tissue is wearing away. Physician-researchers at the University of California believe this happens when the area surrounding the stem cells, called the niche or micro environment, also ages to the point where it affects the stem cell's ability to preserve and repair healthy tissue. They theorize that if they can slow the pace of aging in the niche, they will be able to find new ways to transform these micro environments so that they can help the body's existing stem cells perform better.

In a study presented at a symposium of The Buck Institute for Research on Aging in 2012, researchers also noted the impact that a stem cell's environment had on the stem cell. They exposed older stem cells to younger ones in a process called Heterochronic Parabiosis, whereby the older stem cells could be stimulated to act like younger ones. The converse was also true. Younger, less stable stem cells benefited from their exposure to more mature cells, helping to make them more stable.

Incidentally, cosmetic surgeons performing liposuction have known for some time that fat is loaded with stem cells. Studies have shown that fat has healing properties as well — properties doctors attributed to the proliferation of stem cells. These doctors learned that fat grafting in mice reverses radiation damage. Within these grafts, hair grew, skin color and texture improved, scar tissue decreased, and vascular density increased. Their study holds important developments for cancer patients undergoing radiation treatment.

In humans, innovative cosmetic surgeons are using fat-grafting to restore a sense of youthfulness in the face in a procedure they informally dub the stem cell facelift. Skin that is fat-grafted not only adds more volume to the hollow areas of the eyes and cheeks, it also lessens wrinkles, and leaves the skin rosier with better texture. Fat-grafting has some benefits over other forms of synthetic collagen (sometimes called fillers). First, the injection is natural, originating from the person's own body. Secondly, the grafted stem cells become self-perpetuating, developing fresh stem cells as people continue to age. This means patients do not need to have continuous fat-grafts in the same area because the stem cells in the grafts are producing more cells and thereby more volume in the face. The first facial fat-graft in the United States was performed in Beverly Hills, California eight years ago and the female recipient continues to appear improved. Had she opted for synthetic collagen treatment instead, doctors would have had to re-inject the material approximately every six months to achieve the same results.

ALS (Lou Gehrig's Disease): Are Clinical Trials Making the Progression from Animals to Humans?

To date, stem cell therapy works well in rats, but is not achieving the desired outcomes in humans. This doesn't mean that human treatment has failed; it means researchers must learn the secret to successfully implanting the healing cells in the human body. In June 2011, physicians in Atlanta, Georgia began safety trials on ALS patients to determine if stem cells could be injected into the spinal cord without adverse effects.

Alzheimer's Disease: What are Potential Keys to Eliminating Alzheimer's?

Alzheimer's robs patients of their memory until they can no longer recall family names and significant life moments. The disease occurs when individuals have too much plaque in their brains. The key to rejuvenation seems to lie in first eliminating the APP plaque cells (Amyloid-Beta-Precursor Proteins), secondly regenerating the dopamine cells, and thirdly replacing the dead neurons. Because there are so many types of nerve cells in the brain, it is challenging to develop therapies for Alzheimer's.

Nevertheless, human neural stem cells have been transplanted into the brains of aged rats and allowed to differentiate into other neural cells. There has been improved cognitive function in the animals. Newer studies take adult mesenchymal stem cells found in bone marrow and allow them to differentiate into neural cells, modifying the DNA so that the cells become similar to those in an embryonic stem cell. Results are pending.

Researchers are also questioning glia's role in improving Alzheimer's. Glia is known as the glue that holds neurons together and one of glia's key properties is that it continues to undergo cell division into adulthood, whereas many neurons do not. When APP protein levels are reduced in the brain during Alzheimer's, glia stem cell differentiation is also reduced. When glia cells proliferate, there is an improvement in the regeneration of neurons.

Autism: Does Hope Lie in Stem Cells from the Umbilical Cord?

Like cancer, autism is actually a group of disorders with many different factors that can affect the results. Sometimes there are inflammatory aspects to the disease; then too, it is possible that the disease strikes because too little blood reaches the brain and the nerve cells. Stem cell therapies for autism have been marketed, but there is little scientific documentation that they actually work. New hope lies in stem cell therapies using umbilical cord blood.

In August 2012, researchers at Sutter Medical Center in Sacramento, California initiated a clinical trial for autistic children, ages 2 to 7, using stem cells banked from their own umbilical cords. This marked the first time a clinical trial had been approved for autism by the Food and Drug Administration, modeled after FDA approved clinical trials for cerebral palsy. The trial monitors autistic patients for improvements in language and behavior.

Favorable results have been documented when treatment for autism has been sought outside the United States. An infant living in Maine was diagnosed with autism at age two. As a 7-year-old child, he couldn't talk; at age 8, he couldn't read. In 2009, his parents took him to Costa Rica for pioneering stem cell treatment using stem cells from umbilical cord blood. Within days of treatment, the boy's parents noticed improvements. A year later, their son could read, speak with sentence structure, remember birthdays, and tell time. Network television reported on the child's story nationally, giving hope to many.

Autoimmune Diseases: Years After Studies Began, is there a Track Record in Human Trials?

A study from the University of Basel in Switzerland tracked approximately 1,500 patients who received hematopoietic stem cell therapies for autoimmune diseases including Multiple Sclerosis, Lupus, Rheumatoid Arthritis, Systemic Sclerosis or Scleroderma, ITP, and Juvenile Arthritis. More than a third of those in the study were MS or Systemic Sclerosis patients. At the five-year mark, 85% of patients had survived their diseases and 43% had no further progression of their diseases.

Bone Marrow Transplants: What is a Bone Marrow Transplant?

Bone marrow transplants have become familiar in the treatment of cancers such as leukemia and lymphoma. Many people do not realize that a bone marrow transplant is actually a stem cell transplant.

Even though the first bone marrow transplants were performed in the 1959, they remain very drastic measures today and they are difficult for the patient to endure. With autologous bone marrow transplants, stem cells from the patient's bone marrow are extracted, treated, and saved for later use. Then, although it leaves the patient completely unprotected from infection or disease, every cell in the body is destroyed through chemotherapy and radiation therapy, concentrating first on the areas where cancer cells multiply quickly. Once every cell is destroyed, doctors work quickly to reintroduce specially treated stem cells back into the patient, encouraging cells to repopulate the bone marrow. If the bone marrow transplant is successful, these cells live and continue to multiply.

Cancer: What New Paths of Discovery are Researchers Following?

The California Institute for Regenerative Medicine (CIRM) has initiated a study that uses human gene therapy to treat melanoma. Melanoma, which is more rampant in areas with plenty of sun, has been increasing by 15% over the last decade. Researchers use human embryonic stem cells and hematopoietic stem cells to produce new cells that are able to kill human melanoma in petri dishes. The study now advances to the animal testing stage. If successful, researchers will be able to create gene therapy that will destroy cancerous melanoma tumors.

In order for healthy human immune systems to work, they must maintain a delicate balance; they must guard an individual from harmful disease, all the while refrain from negatively attacking the body's own tissue. Scientists are experimenting with Dendritic Cells (DC) — cells in the immune system that naturally search for and attach themselves to antigens in the body in order to fight disease. Experimentation works like this: once a tumor is removed from the body, scientists search for a cancer stem cell within it; their goal is to use it to make a vaccine-like injection that will contain enough of the cancer to cause immunity, but not enough to cause disease. Once reintroduced into the body, the antigens in the injection tackle the cancer, leaving normal cells intact. This new way of thinking is a huge departure from procedures like traditional bone marrow transplants, where all of the patient's cells are destroyed before reintroducing healthy, cancer-free cells.

The delicate equilibrium in healthy immune systems becomes even more precarious as doctors transplant stem cells from one individual to another. At CIRM, researchers are experimenting with DC cells that recognize stem cells from one donor and react as if they were those of the patient. Researchers are encouraged by DC cells which could allow stem cell grafts from patient to patient go more smoothly, without rejection.

Researchers in Singapore are also experimenting with DC cells derived from embryonic stem cells in humans, in hopes of developing economical vaccines for cancer that may eventually become available over the counter. Meanwhile, The US Food and Drug Administration has approved its first DC-based vaccine prepared from a patient's own body; to date, this is an expensive process that has produced variable results in clinical trials, however.

Scientists at the University of Michigan have been studying the stem cells in cancer for a decade, in virtually every type of tumor, but especially in pancreatic cancer, and cancer of the head and neck. They believe cancer treatment sometimes fails because the stem cells in cancer are not destroyed. Other discoveries at its Cancer Center have determined that mutations in certain genes encourage breast cancer cells to divide and renew quickly, invading nearby breast tissue with devastating results. Drugs inhibiting these genes reduced the number of stem cells in cancer. In addition, doctors have identified a receptor on the surface of the cancer stem cells that activates abnormal cell growth when receptors are exposed to inflammation and the damage caused by chemo-therapy. Blocking the receptor prevents the cancer from spreading.

More than a dozen years after experimental treatment began, Stanford researchers have obtained statistics that show women with metastatic breast cancer, who are treated to *both* high dose chemotherapy followed by a transplant of their own blood-forming stem cells, are more likely to survive. Chemo destroys the cancer but it also obliterates the patient's bone marrow, which is responsible for producing blood and immune cells. Doctors found that if they removed some of the patient's bone marrow before the chemo began, then purified the stem cells before re-injecting it back into the patient, there was lesser chance that the re-injected blood cells would develop into cancer cells. After surveying patients, Stanford researchers found 23 percent of the women from the original study were still alive; compared to 9 percent whose therapy did not include the blood-forming stem cells.

Standard (cytotoxic) chemotherapy has been ineffective in treating malignant gliomas, a type of brain tumor. Surgery and radiation have not been successful combatants either, because glioma tumor cells are constantly on the move throughout the brain's territory, evading the therapy. However, some types of stem cells do gravitate toward tumor cells regardless of where they are located in the brain. Researchers are experimenting with these stem cells, trying to employ genetic engineering that seeks out the tumor cells and destroys them. At City of Hope near Los Angeles, testing has produced positive results in animals.

Cerebral Palsy: Are Therapies Showing Promise in the Betterment of Motor Skills?

For every 1,000 children born, approximately two to three are diagnosed with cerebral palsy, a neurological disease that impedes verbal and physical growth that is often caused by brain injuries occurring at birth due to oxygen deprivation. Researchers at the Department of Neurosurgery and Stanford Stroke Center have been injecting genetically-engineered human neural stem cells into animals, along with a method for tracking them. After twenty four hours, researchers found human neural stem cells grafted onto the forebrain of the animals. Four weeks later, the rats showed improved movement of their forelimbs, suggesting that human neural stem cell transplants were promising for children born with cerebral palsy.

In a human trial, researchers injected stem cells into the spinal cavity of patient, where blood vessels supply the brain with blood and oxygen. After one year, patients in this trial exceeded their earlier abilities in movement and coordination. Just as importantly, no one showed signs of complications from the stem cell injections.

Still, in other research conducted on cerebral palsy patients, doctors experimented with patients' previously banked cord blood which had been intravenously infused with stem cell-rich cryopreserved blood. Patients in this trial, who were once unable to move corresponding parts on both sides of their bodies, saw significant improvement in this motor skill; so did patients who were totally or partially immobile on one side. Quadriplegics, however, saw little improvement in this study.

Diabetes I and II:

While researchers have shown that human embryonic stem cells can be differentiated into pancreatic progenitors (which are like stem cells in their ability to divide and restore, but are more highly differentiated than stem cells), they must also develop a controlled and regulated process to manufacture these cells in order to treat Type I Diabetes. Doctors in Athens, Georgia are experimenting with ways to expand and bank the differentiated cells, but also to form an integrated manufacturing process capable of mass producing pancreatic progenitors. They have successfully developed a virtually unlimited supply of single cells that begin a four-stage protocol that ultimately determines pancreatic cell lines. Islet-like tissue from this process containing insulin-secreting cells has been implanted in mice for study.

Meanwhile in Brussels, when mouse islet cells were cultured with neural crest stem cells, researchers created a new in vitro system that lead to their own increased production of islet beta cells. The cells were fully glucose responsive in their insulin secretion capabilities.

In Israel, researchers are trying to develop the best conditions for generating and isolating cells for transplantation therapy. They have turned to stem cell-derived progenitor cells from the pancreas that have the ability to become insulin-producing cells; first by identifying, isolating and characterizing each stage of the progenitor cells; then by specifically identifying novel molecules in the process of differentiation as well as stage-specific markers.

Even researchers in India are intent on finding a cure for Diabetes using the potential of progenitor cells to expand human islets-derived progenitor cells.

Other studies hope to cure Diabetes through mesenchymal stem cell infusions. Researchers have shown that these infusions can play multiple roles in improving Type II Diabetes. It had been previously established that these injections were capable of lowering blood glucose levels in diabetic patients. A study involving diabetic rats has now shown that mesenchymal stem cell injections improve insulin sensitivity as well.

Mesenchymal stem cells in the human umbilical cord and placenta are under study for their potential role in differentiating into functional islets that can be transplanted into diabetic patients.

Emphysema:

Chronic obstructive pulmonary disease (COPD) occurs when there are vascular changes in the pulmonary (lung) or other circulatory systems in the body resulting from a reduction in blood and vascular progenitors. Bone marrow has the ability to produce progenitor cells that may be used in areas where vascular damage has occurred.

Therefore, stem cell regeneration is a promising solution for controlling respiratory diseases, although studies are still in early stages: lungs are the most challenging organ to regenerate.

It should be noted that some Italian researchers are taking a cautionary approach to stem cells as a therapy for COPD. They believe that more translational studies must be performed before clinical trials advance. More information is necessary about cells subsets, they believe, insisting that deadly neoplasms are a possible result from stem cells.

There is evidence in mice and circumstantial evidence in humans, however, that Acute Respiratory Distress Syndrome prompts lung tissue to regenerate. Using stem cells from this lung tissue, researchers have created cloned human airway stem cells in vitro.

Meanwhile, mesenchymal stem cell therapy has been applied in the trachea of rats with chronic pulmonary disease. Improvement in their conditions also showed a significant change in proteome levels. During this study, more than 300 lung proteins were identified and documented. The results suggested that protein-based tissue may be the key to improving COPD.

Other studies have confirmed that mesenchymal stem cells produce positive results in lung development, repair, and remodeling. Grafting of an injured lung does not occur easily, but the therapy produces less inflammation as it promotes the repair of tissue. More study is needed, but researchers are optimistic that stem cell therapy can improve respiratory diseases.

Heart Attacks & Heart Damage: Are Small Steps Laying the Foundation for True Advancements?

While there have been important scientific breakthroughs in this area, the heart is a complicated organ and much must still be accomplished before real solutions are safely possible. Every day the news becomes more encouraging, however. Researchers conducting a small study using human patients at Cedars-Sinai Heart Institute in Los Angeles have dissolved scar tissue and replaced it with living heart muscle, using stem cells and minimally invasive procedures. From a limited number of stem cells obtained from each patient, researchers generated 12-25 million new stem cells and transplanted them back into their respective patients. One year later, scar tissue in the transplant area had shrunk by about 50%, increasing the area of live heart tissue. The procedure reduced the overall size of the heart, but researchers are still trying to understand how to make the improved heart pump blood more efficiently.

When a company employs researchers all over the world, it has the ability to perform clinical trials — and gain knowledge — that might be restricted in the U.S. Cytori Therapeutics, headquartered in San Diego, California is such a company. In the U.S., Cytori is conducting safety and feasibility trials for refractory heart failure, a condition that occurs when the heart cannot produce enough blood for the body to sustain itself adequately. As a result, shortness of breath, palpitations, swelling of the legs, and even an enlarged heart can occur. However in Europe, Cytori has advanced beyond the gathering of safety and feasibility studies to human double-blind clinical trials that seek to reduce the size of blood clots in the coronary artery, therefore reducing the potential for heart attack.

HIV: Have Researchers Found a Cure for AIDS?

A 45-year-old man known as 'the Berlin Patient', had been deemed the first person 'cured' of AIDS. Timothy Ray Brown, a United States citizen residing in Berlin at the time, had been treated for both Leukemia and AIDS. Doctors performed a bone marrow transplant using rare stem cells from another donor featuring a lack of the CCR5 receptor, a mutation that appears in less than 1% of Caucasians in Europe. Once the diseased cells had been removed and the donor's cells transplanted in their place, Brown was taken off anti-viral drugs. After surviving five years, he was deemed HIV-free. In July 2012, Brown spoke before the International AIDS conference in Washington, D.C., where he stated that he remained HIV-negative. At the conference, a doctor from the University of California expressed some doubts about this claim. The doctor had tested tissues from Brown's blood cells, plasma, and rectum, which showed some evidence of HIV; however, the doctor also admitted that it was uncertain if the evidence was real or the result of contamination.

Clearly, this case showed that bone marrow transplants were (and they still are), considered drastic protocols for treating AIDS; additionally the limited availability of the transplanted stem cells and the exorbitant cost of treatment make this an unlikely cure for the overall HIV-infected population. Whether the Berlin Patient's HIV-free status holds up or not, stem cells have played an important role in eradicating the disease.

What Do Researchers Hope to Learn About?

Liver Damage

Researchers at the Okohama City University Graduate School of Medicine in Japan have created liver "buds" from induced pluripotent stem cells, generating new hope that full size liver organs may one day be derived in the lab for human transplant (or) that miniature livers may be cultivated from the skin cells of dying patients and used to improve their existing liver function. The 2013 discovery combined three types of human liver cells in the lab, which not only survived, but grew into the three-dimensional structures the researchers called "buds". Once transplanted into mice, human blood vessels inside the buds connected to the mouse blood vessels and began functioning much like mature human liver cells. If all goes well, scientists speculate that the development of a full scale human liver organ is at least ten years away. More immediately however, the buds could be used to develop promising new drugs to aid liver function.

Macular Degeneration

Scientists have injected human embryonic stem cells into the eyes of patients in both the United States and Japan, showing promising results in the treatment of macular degeneration. The safety and tolerability study at UCLA and Advanced Cell Technology in Massachusetts was small and more studies are needed, but the initial study involving a woman with Stargardt's macular dystrophy, and another with macular degeneration caused by age, saw both patients experiencing improved vision.

Additionally, Japanese researchers have been given approval to conduct trials that aim to regenerate the retinas of patients. Using skin cells converted into pluripotent stem cells, researchers plan to allow the cells to differentiate into a layer of the retina that would then be transplanted onto human retinas and allowed to graft. The next stage of the trials will monitor the stem cells' ability to improve vision. Trials are expected to begin in 2014.

Multiple Sclerosis (MS)

The Cleveland Clinic has begun a Phase I clinical trial using the mesenchymal stem cells found in bone marrow to treat, and perhaps even reverse, MS. Researchers collected approximately 70 million of the cells, the amount needed for a 150 pound man, from a patient's own bone marrow. Once cultivated, they were infused intravenously back into his arm. Doctors acknowledge it will take time to determine if the transplanted stem cells impacted the patient's health. The Cleveland Clinic trial is one of four sites to conduct the MS Phase I trials. Other hospitals are in Spain and Iran. Meanwhile, other countries have begun recruiting patients for a study using mesenchymal stem cells as treatment for MS.

Muscular Dystrophy

Treatment for muscular dystrophy has been hampered in the past as researchers found it difficult to use embryonic stem cells and induced pluripotent stem cells to create muscle cells. Scientists at the University of Minnesota Lillehei Heart Institute have now isolated an effective process that efficiently pushes these stem cells into forming human muscle progenitor cells. By using the PAX7 gene and addressing the PAX7 protein, researchers have been able to coax stem cells into differentiating into muscle-forming cells more abundantly.

In addition, researchers at Purdue University have found that controlling the oxygen levels of stem cells produced in a petri dish before implanting them in mice, allows more of the transplanted stem cells to survive. The discovery hinged on regulating oxygen levels so that they were more aligned with levels found in the human body. Initially, researchers were able to produce more muscle-differentiated stem cells at the higher level of oxygen, but the cells frequently did not survive.

Children with the specific form of Duchenne Muscular Dystrophy often fail to reach adulthood because of heart and breathing complications. Researchers have been trying to understand why, but found that lab mice bearing the same Duchenne genetic mutation as the children, showed only mild MD symptoms without the cardiac disability. Doctors at Stanford University School of Medicine have finally engineered mice that accurately simulate the children's form of the disease. The length of the telomeres at the ends of the chromosomes was cited as the factor.

Osteoarthritis & Osteoporosis

Repairing a bone fracture or replacing a hip may one day be successful thanks to the use of a degradable plastic honeycomb-style implant. Researchers theorize that the implant attracts the stem cells in bone marrow and encourages new bone formation, which replaces the implant over time. Development is still in the lab stage but has been tested in animals with promising results. The research is a joint collaboration of the University of Southampton, United Kingdom; the University of Glasgow, Scotland; and the University of Edinburgh, Scotland.

In a related study in Malaysia, one doctor has successfully treated more than 200 patients by micro-drilling small holes in the bone of the knee at the site of damaged cartilage. The surgery is followed by several weekly injections of a stem cell-rich blood product created from the patient's body. These cells are capable of differentiating into healthy cartilage. The doctor theorizes that the drilling creates a blood clot scaffolding — a base to add substance — as the blood product attaches to it. When hyaluronic acid is added, it generates better cartilage as well as less pain for the patient. The procedure works even in difficult bone-on-bone cartilage damaged cases.

Parkinson's Disease

Doctors already know that a specific type of nerve cell within the brain is affected during Parkinson's Disease — and that the cells die and can no longer produce the dopamine that is necessary to control tremors like those seen in the disease's most famous patient, actor Michael J. Fox. Parkinson's also causes some people to lose their sense of smell and/or have sleep disorders. As the disease progresses, they may even suffer from dementia. Scientists think it may be possible to treat Parkinson's by replacing the lost cells with new ones. They are already using stem cells in the lab to grow new nerve cells. Researchers from Sweden, Canada, and America have successfully transplanted dopamine-producing neurons (nerve cells) from fetuses into other patients, but their work has produced inconsistent results. Ultimately, the goal is to introduce new cells that could delay the onset or advancement of Parkinson's. Researchers acknowledge however, that beyond the ethical barriers of using embryonic stem cells, enough embryonic tissue simply doesn't exist to care for the large Parkinson's population. In 2010, U.S. scientists began experimenting with induced pluripotent stem cells (IPS) made from adult skin cells, transplanting them into the brain. The procedure in rats showed promise, but more studies are needed to explore the long term safety for human use.

Furthermore, at the Buck Institute for Research on Aging symposium held in March 2012 in Novato, California, it was noted that a four-year clinical trial injecting fetal brain stem cells into adult patients with Parkinson's produced unfavorable side effects and outcomes. It was thought that perhaps the results would have been more promising had the patients' illnesses not progressed to the dyskinesia movement disorder stage of the disease. To complicate matters, with Parkinson's, there can be significant loss of communication between nerve cells at the synaptic junction before the disease is even detected. The synapse allows neurons to transmit messages from cell to cell and without it, it is more difficult for newly injected stem cells to communicate with the cell environment.

Spinal Cord Injury

Early findings in a randomized trial conducted in New Jersey indicate that when patients with cervical or thoracic spinal cord injuries are treated with both physical therapy and stem cell therapy, they respond better on the AIS (American Spinal Injury Impairment Scale) than patients who receive only physical therapy. At the University of Medicine and Dentistry of New Jersey — Robert Wood Johnson Medical School, the first phase of the trial consisted of 70 patients divided into two groups. The group that was injected with stem cells from their own bone marrow saw sensory or motor functions improve, while the control group that lacked exposure to stem cells did not. Some injected patients saw rapid improvement in their tactile and sensory responses — appearing as early as four weeks. By twelve weeks patients gained muscle strength which produced better bladder and bowel control; eventually they were able to discard their catheters. After a year and a half, nearly half of the stem cell recipients saw a 10 point improvement on the AIS (American Spinal Injury Impairment Scale) and some were even able to walk with assistance. Those with thoracic spinal cord injuries showed the most gain.

A small trial at the Spinal Cord Injury Center at Balgrist University Hospital, University of Zurich has shown optimistic results in patients who have the worst kind of injury to the spinal cord. It is the first time that neural stem cells were transplanted during stem cell therapy. Two of the three patients gained significant sensory capabilities. Although the goal of the trial was to determine the safety of neural stem cell transplantation, the doctors were encouraged to discover the degree of improvement. Patients had suffered complete injury to the chest area (thoracic spinal cord) and had been left paralyzed below the injury. Twenty million stem cells were injected at the site of damage. The patients' gain in sensitivity involved changes in touch, heat, and electrical stimuli in specific areas below the level of injury. Additionally, the patients' sensory capabilities remained constant. A third patient, however, showed no signs of improvement. Continuation of the trial will monitor changes in sensation, as well as motor function and bowel/bladder function. After completion of the trial, long-term observation of the participants is planned.

Stroke

In more than 80% of strokes, the stroke occurs because a blocked artery makes it impossible for the normal flow of oxygen and blood to get to the brain. This destroys approximately two million brain cells every minute the stroke continues. Researchers are experimenting with a genetically engineered stem cell therapy that has the potential to enhance motor skills after a stroke, and it is derived from an adult donor's own bone marrow. The cells are transferred into the brain near the damage and appear to stimulate the brain to heal itself. The process has worked well in animals and trials have begun in humans. The study is a combined effort between Northwestern University Feinberg School of Medicine, the University of Pittsburgh Medical Center, and Stanford University School of Medicine.

In Glasgow, a small study of six stroke patients has documented improvement in the mobility of the patients' limbs and one patient has even regained the ability to speak after being treated with the stem cells of a twelve-week old fetus. The results surprised researchers of the Institute of Neurological Sciences at the Southern General Hospital, who had injected the stem cells into the brains of the patients in a safety study, but who were encouraged to learn of the overall progress. The patients were participating in the trial after having suffered their strokes from six months to five years prior. Further trials will be necessary to determine if the stem cells actually repaired the damaged brains.

Epilogue
Tony V. Lu, M.D.

Untangling the Controversy . . .

I am, first and foremost, a clinician. Throughout my medical career, I have been both a lab bench technician and a clinical doctor who must sometimes break difficult news to my patients. Experiences that have been both professionally fulfilling and yet sometimes personally agonizing have shaped the way I view the potential of stem cell exploration — and I suppose that automatically creates a bias in my reasoning. Nonetheless, I have tried to present you with the information you need to come to your own ideas about this fascinating and still developing area of medicine, without bullying you to come to the same conclusions I hold. Mostly I hope to encourage you to ask the next question so that your curiosities might challenge the future of stem cell research. This book has been written simply so that if you are a patient who desires to speak to a doctor about hopeful new medical strategies, you will have the basic understanding of stem cells and what might be possible to help heal you. If you are an up and coming physician — or even a well-seasoned one who has never had a reason to be closely associated with this remarkable area of study — I hope to entice you to learn more about it, possibly even adding a new direction to your career.

I have enjoyed presenting these scientific and social aspects of stem cell exploration to you. Before ending this book, I thought you might like to know some of my closely held beliefs about stem cell research and all its potential.

I am a naturalized citizen of the United States and have been for thirty plus years. I went to college in Seattle and attended medical school in New York; I have lived in the U.S. for a total of 38 years, but have also studied and worked in other countries before returning here to care for United States Veterans from Vietnam, Iraq and Afghanistan. What those like me who are born outside the democracy of the States most admire in this country are its citizens' rights to consider alternative points of view. There will always be those with religious or political convictions that do not honor the exploration of science when it concerns human creation — and I respect that. But I also know that until one is confronted with a no-hope or tragic disease, they have not witnessed the sheer panic felt by a patient or parent of a patient whose life has been threatened. Nancy Reagan changed her mind about stem cell research after experiencing President Reagan's Alzheimer Disease first hand. I don't believe that her heartfelt change in view is a fault in character. I believe it is the result of a loving human being who is trying to address the unimaginable truth of disease. The desire to live is so strong in all of us. To those who have never faced medical trauma, I hope you never have to and I understand your need to hold on to your convictions. If you do not believe in stem cell medicine, it is your prerogative to forego its current uses and many advances. However, when someone is sick and is looking for a medical miracle, I encourage you to put your personal convictions aside, and support their need to find such a miracle.

As for stem cell's intrusive ability to potentially alter the future of the human body, any scientist would tell you that every solidified, proven, and reliable aspect to modern day living once faced the uncertainty of the unknown. We know that before Columbus sailed the seas, the earth was thought to be flat and that a daily diet of meat and potatoes was once thought to be healthy. Today open heart surgery, in-vitro fertilization, and even bone marrow transplants can still be dangerous, but we accept them and pray for them to take hold when the need is dire. Extreme circumstances require extreme answers. When the residents of Hiroshima, Japan were affected by radiation poisoning during World War II, many would have lived if they had been able to obtain antidotal treatment. In this century, our world is once again as dangerous. The attack on human life is both widespread in the case of terrorism and war, but also personal in the more intimate cases of individualized murder. As danger evolves, so too must our remedies. I agree with the many other researchers who believe the safest medical treatments will one day originate from our own bodies. In the severest of developments, it may be all we can rely on!

Will commerce eventually be responsible for the widespread manufacturing of stem cell products — and control their availabilities through supply and demand, sometimes with financial constraints? This should not be surprising; in fact, it should be expected. This is the way healthcare works in the United States. That little blue pill you take as well as your blood pressure medicine has become readily available at the prescription counter because an enterprising company chose to fund the research and market the successes. Next to federal funding, big businesses are the largest contributors to scientific research. Their contributions make it possible for us to put wondrous new products in your hands. I believe that innovative new procedures in stem cell research should be tested and regulated before coming to market, but I also believe that it is possible to tie researchers' hands in over-regulation so that nothing new can develop. The key to research, development, and marketing lies in honoring a reasonable balance.

As for stem cell's closely debated association with abortion, on one hand, I wish this never had happened. Researchers in the United States lost 8 valuable years in our ability to bring new cures to fruition, years other countries did not. It gave countries like Germany and China new footholds in scientific development that will come back to haunt the United States as it struggles to retain world leadership status on so many levels. If ever something good could come out of something bad, however, the abortion debate was responsible for one thing. It challenged researchers to find another avenue to stem cell creation beyond the use of embryonic stem cells. Once scientists figured out how to create induced pluripotent stem cells that had the characteristics of embryonic stem cells but could be accessed from adult stem cells — found as commonplace as those on a person's arm — a whole new universe opened up in stem cell's possibilities.

Will stem cell innovation coupled with genetic engineering and gene cloning be the end all and cure all for disease? That's a nice thought, but probably not. More likely, researchers have stumbled upon the next important step that will offer great solutions in preventing and curing aging and disease. Stem cells will be but the next Eureka moment in medical history upon which the next Eureka moments will be built.

Bibliography

Preface:

In 2012, John B. Gurdon and Shinya Yamanaka were jointly honored
Nobel Prize. "The 2012 Nobel Prize in Physiology or Medicine - Press Release."
Accessed November 26, 2012.
http://www.nobelprize.org/nobel_prizes/medicine/laureates/2012/press.html.

Chapter 1:

Tuskegee Study

In return for participating in the publicly funded study
Encyclopedia of Alabama. "Tuskegee Syphilis Study."
Accessed November 28, 2012
http://www.encyclopediaofAlabama.org/face/Article.jsp?id+h-1116.

When the men underwent more complex testing
"Tuskegee Syphilis Study."

Doctors believed the biggest contribution
"Tuskegee Syphilis Study."

They were only informed they had bad blood
Centers for Disease Control and Prevention. "The Tuskegee Timeline."
Accessed August 13, 2012.
http://www.cdc.gov/tuskegee/timeline.html.

It was halted in 1972
"The Tuskegee Timeline."

HeLa Cells

Skloot, Rebecca. *The Immortal Life of Henrietta Lacks.*
Broadway Paperbacks/Crown Publishing Group. 2010, 2011.

Rebecca Skloot. "About The Immortal Life of Henrietta Lacks."
Accessed August 14, 2012.
http: http://rebeccaskloot.com/the-immortal-life/.

Smithsonian. "Henrietta Lacks' 'Immortal' Cells."
Accessed August 14, 2012.
www.smithsonianmag.com/science-nature/Henrietta-Lacks-Immortal-Cells.html.

Monsanto

Robert Kenner. *Food, Inc.* (Documentary). 2008.

Vanity Fair. "Monsanto's Harvest of Fear."
Accessed December 17, 2012.
http://www.vanityfair.com/politics/features/2008/05/monsanto200805.

By 2006, nearly 2,400 farmers
Christian Science Monitor. "Control over your food: Why Monsanto's GM seeds are undemocratic."
Accessed September 13, 2012.
http://www.csmonitor.com/Commentary/Opinion/2011/0223/Control-over-your-food-Why...

During a 15-year period, only 145 lawsuits
Monsanto. "Settling the Matter."
Accessed December 17, 2012.
http:// www.monsanto.com/newsviews/Pages/settling-the-matter-part-5.aspx.

At one point, the Center for Food Safety
"Control over your food: Why Monsanto's GM seeds are undemocratic."

However, there have also been complaints
Vanity Fair. "How Seed Giant Monsanto Went from 2009 Company of the Year to Worst Stock of 201."
Accessed December 17, 2012.
http://www.vanityfair.com/online/daily/2010/10/how-seed-giant-monsanto-went-from-20...

Chapter 2:

The Charismatic Stem Cell

Background Research:
EuroStemCell. "Embryonic stem cells: where do they come from and what can they do?"
Accessed July 26, 2012.
http://www.eurostemcell.org/factsheet/embryonic-stem-cells-where-do-they-come-and-wh...

National Institute of Health. "Stem Cell Basics I."
Accessed July 25, 2012
http://stemcells.nih.gov/info/basics/basics1.asp.

National Institute of Health. "Stem Cell Basics II."
Accessed July 25, 2012
http://stemcells.nih.gov/info/basics/basics2.asp.

National Institute of Health. "Stem Cell Basics III."
Accessed July 25, 2012
http://stemcells.nih.gov/info/basics/basics3.asp.

National Institute of Health. "Stem Cell Basics IV."
Accessed July 25, 2012
http://stemcells.nih.gov/info/basics/basics4.asp.

National Institute of Health. "Stem Cell Basics V."
Accessed July 25, 2012
http://stemcells.nih.gov/info/basics/basics5.asp.

National Institute of Health. "Stem Cell Basics VI."
Accessed July 25, 2012
http://stemcells.nih.gov/info/basics/basics6.asp.

National Institute of Health. "Bone Marrow (Hematopoietic) Stem Cells."
Accessed August 9, 2012.
http://stemcells.nih.gov/StemCells/Templates/StemCellContentPage.aspx?N
RMODE=Publi...

NOVA. "Stem Cells: Early Research (Video)." Posted April 19, 2004.
Accessed December 3, 2012.
http://www.pbs.org/wgbh/nova/body/stem-cells-research.html.

What Is a Stem Cell?
Tony Lu, MD, personal correspondence to Karen McLaren, July 25, 2012.

Are Humans the Only Species to Have Stem Cells?
Tony Lu, MD, personal correspondence to Karen McLaren, July 25, 2012.

Are There Different Kinds of Human Stem Cells?
Tony Lu, MD, personal correspondence to Karen McLaren, July 25, 2012.

What Are Embryonic Stem Cells?
Tony Lu, MD, personal correspondence to Karen McLaren August 3, 2012.

... and in More Detail?
Medical Textbooks Revealed. "Chapter 1: How Does an Embryo Form?"
http://medicaltextbooksrevealed.com

National Institute of Health. "Stem Cell Basics II."
Accessed July 25, 2012
http://stemcells.nih.gov/info/basics/basics5.asp.

What Are Adult Stem Cells?
National Institute of Health. "Chapter 4: The Adult Stem Cell."
Accessed August 2, 2012.
http://www.Stemcells.nih.gov/info/scireport/chapter4.asp .

Tony Lu, MD, personal correspondence to Karen McLaren August 3, 2012.

What Is The Physical Makeup of a Stem Cell?
Brown University. "Physical properties predict stem cell outcome."
Posted May 21, 2012.
http://news.brown.edu/pressreleases/2012/05/stemcells.

Where Do You Find Stem Cells?
National Institute of Health. "Chapter 4: The Adult Stem Cell."
Accessed April 8, 2012.
http://www.Stemcells.nih.gov/info/scireport/chapter4.asp .

How Are Adult Stem Cells Extracted from the Body?
Tony Lu, MD, personal correspondence to Karen McLaren, July 25, 2012.
Tony Lu, MD, personal correspondence to Karen McLaren, August 10, 2012.

Do Adult Stem Cells Exist in Fat?
UCLA. "UCLA Newsroom: A New Way to Make Bone: Fresh, Purified Fat
Stem Cells Grow Bone Faster, Better."
Accessed August 2, 2012.
http://Newsroom.ucla.edu/portal/ucla/a-better-way-to-grow-bone-fresh-2349
86/aspx.

Tony Lu, MD, personal correspondence to Karen McLaren, August 10, 2012.

Are Doctors Transferring Harvested Fat Stem Cells ...?
UCLA. "A New Way to Make Bone; Fresh, Purified Fat Stem Cells Grow Bone
Faster, Better."
Accessed August 2, 2012.
http://www.newsroom.ucla.edu/portal/ucla/a-better-way-to-grow-bone-fresh-
234986.aspx.

Where Do Doctors Find Risk Takers ...?
Sports News First. "Stem Cell Bid to Save Bartram's Career."
Posted August 2, 2012.
http://www.sportsnewsfirst.com.au/articles/2012/08/02/stem-cell-bid-to-save
-bartram-s-career/

Pigskin Report. "Peyton Manning and Terrell Owens Have Controversial Stem-Cell Therapy Overseas."
Posted September 21, 2011.
http://www.thepigskinreport.com/2011/09/peyton-manning-and-terrell-owens-have-contr

USA Today. "Report: Terrell Owens in South Korea for Treatment."
Posted September 20, 2011.
http://content.usatoday.com/communities/thehuddle/post/2011/09/report-terrell-owns-in-

Where Do Research Stem Cells Come From?
Tony Lu, MD, personal correspondence to Karen McLaren, August 10, 2012.

If I Were Pregnant … Healthier Start in Life?
Tony Lu, MD, personal correspondence to Karen McLaren, July 25, 2012.

Can Adult Stem Cells be Extracted from a Baby's Umbilical Cord?
Tony Lu, MD, personal correspondence to Karen McLaren, July 25, 2012.

What More Would I Want to Know …?
Tony Lu, MD, personal correspondence to Karen McLaren, July 25, 2012.

Should I Make Use of the Banking Option?
Tony Lu, MD, personal correspondence to Karen McLaren, July 25, 2012.

Why?
Tony Lu, MD, personal correspondence to Karen McLaren, August 10, 2012.

How Can We Be Certain the Stem Cells Belong to My Baby?
Tony Lu, MD, personal correspondence to Karen McLaren, August 20, 2012.
Tony Lu, MD, personal correspondence to Karen McLaren, August 29, 2012.

Do Our Body's Stem Cells Change …?
Zhu, Min. "The Effect of Age on Osteogenic, Adipogenic and Proliferative Potential of Female Adipose-Derived Stem Cells." *Journal of Tissue Engineering & Regenerative Medicine*. March 24 2009; 290-301.

Can a Person's Stem Cells Be Transferred Successfully...?
Cryo-Save. "General Questions: Can My Baby's Stem Cells Also be used for Another Family Member?
Accessed May 3, 2013.
http://www.cryo-save.com/bh/en/faq.html

Could Acquiring Younger Stem Cells ...?
Tony Lu, MD, personal correspondence to Karen McLaren, August 29, 2012.

Once Stem Cells Are Introduced in a Body, Can They Be Rejected?
Tony Lu, MD, personal correspondence to Karen McLaren, July 25, 2012.

Are Some Stem Cells Better to Transplant ...?
Tony Lu, MD, personal correspondence to Karen McLaren, October 11, 2012.

If Stem Cells can become Other Types of cells ...?
Tony Lu, MD, personal correspondence to Karen McLaren, August 10, 2012.

Can a Person get a Benign Tumor ....?
Park, Alice. The Stem Cell Hope. New York: Plume, 2012, 281-282.
Tony Lu, MD. Telephone Interview. October, 12, 2012.

Does Cancer Have Stem Cells?
Tony Lu, MD, personal correspondence to Karen McLaren, August 10, 2012.

Can a Stem Cell Be Turned into a Cancer Cell and Therefore a Weapon?
Tony Lu, MD, personal correspondence to Karen McLaren, July 25, 2012.

Chapter 3:

Giving Stem Cells their Due

What Have We Learned from Hiroshima and Nagasaki?
National Institute of Health. "Bone Marrow (Hematopoietic) Stem Cells; Historical Overview."
Accessed August 9, 2012.
http://stemcells.nih.gov/StemCells/Templates/StemCellContentPage.aspx?N
RMODE=Publi.

Could Stem Cells Have Helped this Situation?
Stem Cell Network. "Stem Cell Timeline."
Accessed September 5, 2012.
http://www.stemcellnetwork.ca/index.php?page=stem-cell-timeline.

What Other Countries Were Involved in Early Stem Cell Research?
Stem Cell Network. "Stem Cell Timeline." Accessed September 5, 2012.
http://www.stemcellnetwork.ca/index.php?page=stem-cell-timeline.

And Now?
How Do Researchers Classify Stem Cells?
Tony Lu, MD, personal correspondence to Karen McLaren, July 25, 2012.

What Are Hematopoietic Stem Cells?
National Institute of Health."Bone Marrow (Hematopoietic) Stem Cells."
Accessed August 9, 2012.
http://stemcells.nih.gov/StemCells/Templates/StemCellContentPage.aspx?N
RMODE=Publi...

Tony Lu, MD, personal correspondence to Karen McLaren, August 3, 2012;
August 10, 2012.

What Are Mesenchymal Stem Cells?
National Institute of Health. "Stem Cell Basics IV." Accessed July 25, 2012.
http://stemcells.nih.gov/info/basics/basics4.asp

National Institute of Health.
Accessed August 9, 2012.
http://www.ncbi.nlm.nih.gov/pmc/articles/PMC2957533 .

Tony Lu, MD, personal correspondence to Karen McLaren, August 3, 2012;
August 10, 2012.

Do Hematopoietic and Mesenchymal Stem Cells Co-exist?
Tony Lu, MD, personal correspondence to Karen McLaren, August 10, 2012.

How Can Scientists tell if a Stem Cell is Hematopoietic or Mesenchymal?
Tony Lu, MD, telephone conversation with Karen McLaren, circa
August-September 2012.

Tony Lu, MD, personal correspondence to Karen McLaren, September 12, 2012.

Do Scientists favor using Hematopoietic or Mesenchymal Stem Cells in their Studies?
Tony Lu, MD, personal correspondence to Karen McLaren, September 14, 2012.

Baer, Patrick C. and Geiger, Helmut. "Adipose-Derived Mesenchymal Stromal/Stem Cells: Tissue Localization, Characterization, and Heterogeneity." Stem Cells International (2012);
Accessed May 8, 2013. doi:10.1155/2012/812693.

What Is a Unipotent Stem Cell?
Park, Alice. *The Stem Cell Hope*. New York: Plume, 2012, 296.

What Are Multipotent Stem Cells?
Park, Alice. *The Stem Cell Hope*. New York: Plume, 2012, 296.

What Are Pluripotent Stem Cells?
Park, Alice. *The Stem Cell Hope*. New York: Plume, 2012, 296.

What Are Induced Pluripotent Stem Cells (iPS)?
Park, Alice. *The Stem Cell Hope*. New York: Plume, 2012, 295.

Do Researchers Study Stem Cells Solely for the Purpose of Preventing Disease?
The Dana Foundation. "High Stakes in Human Stem Cell Research."
Posted July 1, 2000.
www.dana.org.

Do Researchers Clone Diseased Cells?
The Dana Foundation. "High Stakes in Human Stem Cell Research."
Posted July 1, 2000.
www.dana.org.

NOVA. "NOVA/Stem Cells: Early Research."
Video posted Nov. 4, 2005. Accessed December 3, 2012.
www.pbs.org/wgbh/nova/body/stem-cells-research.html

Why Did a Controversy Erupt Over the Cloning of Embryonic Stem Cells?
Tony Lu, MD, personal correspondence to Karen McLaren, July 25, 2012.

How Do These Parents Justify the Seemingly Conflicting Views?
PBS. "NOVA/Stem Cells: Early Research." Video posted Nov. 4, 2005.
Accessed December 3, 2013.
http://www.pbs.org/wgbh/nova/body/stem-cells-research.html
Accessed December 3, 2012.

What Are Stem Cell Lines?
Wikipedia. "Stem Cell Line." Accessed May 6, 2012.
http://en.wikipedia.org/wiki/Stem_cell_line.

Tony Lu, MD, personal correspondence to Karen McLaren, October 5, 2012.

What Are the Often-Referenced 60 Embryonic Stem Cell Lines?
CNN. "Inside Politics: President George W. Bush's Address on Stem Cell
Research." Posted August 9, 2001.
http://archives.cnn.com/2001/ALLPOLITICS/09/09/bush.transcript/index.html.

Why Weren't Researchers Content to Experiment on 60 Lines?
Phys.org. "Bush embryonic stem cell lines different from newly derived cell
lines."
Accessed May 1, 2013.
http://phys.org/news/2011-12-bush-embryonic-stem-cell-lines.html#jCp.

Where Did These Lines Originate and Did That Create Problems?
Phys.org. "Bush embryonic stem cell lines different from newly derived cell
lines."
Accessed May 1, 2013.
http://phys.org/news/2011-12-bush-embryonic-stem-cell-lines.html#jCp.

How Many Stem Cell Lines Exist Now?
Erb, Robin, "What U of M is Working to Cure with Stem Cells."
Detroit Free Press, November 18, 2012, 25A.

Who Is Leading the Way in the Registration of Stem Cell Lines?
National Institute of Health. "Grants & Funding."
Accessed May 8, 2013.
http://GRANTS.NIH.GOV/STEM_CELLS/REGISTRY/CURRENT.HTM.

What Is Important About these Stem Cell Lines?
Erb, Robin, "What U of M is Working to Cure with Stem Cells." Detroit Free Press, November 18, 2012, 25A.

Who Has Been a Prominent Funder of Stem Cell Research?
Charlotte Lozier Institute. "The Ethical Stems of Good Science." Accessed December 3, 2012. http://www.lozierinstitute.org.

What Has CIRM Funded?
Charlotte Lozier Institute. "The Ethical Stems of Good Science." Accessed December 3, 2012. http://www.lozierinstitute.org.

Has CIRM Influenced the Direction of Research Based on its Grant Approvals?
Charlotte Lozier Institute. "The Ethical Stems of Good Science." Accessed December 3, 2012. http://www.lozierinstitute.org.

Chapter 4:

Cloning and Stem Cells

Park, Alice. *The Stem Cell Hope*. "Chapter 2: It Began With Dolly." New York: Plume, 2012.

Are Coaxing Stem Cells and Genetic Engineering - One and the Same?
Tony Lu, MD, personal correspondence to Karen McLaren, August 10, 2012.

What Is the Difference, then, Between Coaxing … and Conducting Genetic Engineering?
Tony Lu, MD, personal correspondence to Karen McLaren, August 10, 2012.

Wikipedia. "Genetic Engineering." Accessed September 19, 2012. http://en.wikipedia.org/wiki/Genetic_Engineering.

Are Stem Cell Alteration and Cloning the Same?
Tony Lu, MD, personal correspondence to Karen McLaren, August 10, 2012.

Then What is Cloning?
National Human Genome Research Institute of the NIH. "Cloning Factsheet."
Accessed September 19, 2012.
www.genome.gov/25020028.

Dolly, the First Cloned Adult Mammal,
Park, Alice. *The Stem Cell Hope*. New York: Plume, 2012, 12, 15, 16, 23.

How Did Dolly Come to Be?
Park, Alice. *The Stem Cell Hope*. New York: Plume, 2012, 12, 15, 16, 23.

So How Did Wilmut Clone a Sheep?
Park, Alice. *The Stem Cell Hope*. New York: Plume, 2012, 12, 15, 16, 23.

What Was Dolly's Ultimate Impact on the Science of Stem Cells?
Park, Alice. *The Stem Cell Hope*. New York: Plume, 2012, 12, 15, 16, 23.

What is Reproductive Cloning?
MedicineNet.com. "Definition of Human Reproductive Cloning."
Accessed May 9, 2013.
http://www.medterms.com/script/main/art.asp?articlekey=26133.

What is Therapeutic Cloning?
Park, Alice. *The Stem Cell Hope*. New York: Plume, 2012, 296.

"Wilmut had no interest in generating a herd of sheep ..."
Park, Alice. *The Stem Cell Hope*. New York: Plume, 2012, 21.

But Can't Patients Opt for a Donor Transplant Instead?
U.S. Department of Health and Human Services Office on Women's Health.
"Organ Donation and Transplantation Fact Sheet."
Accessed October 23, 2012.
http://www.womenshealth.gov/publications/our-publications/fact-sheet/organ
-donation.cfm
Accessed October 23, 2012.

When Stem Cells are Cloned, Can They Actually Be Used in Medical Practice?
Tony Lu, MD, personal correspondence to Karen McLaren, January 15, 2013.

Where Do Other Countries Stand in Their Stem Cell Capabilities?
Science Progress. "China's Recipe for Stem Cell Success."
Accessed February 6, 2013.
http://scienceprogress.org/2010/-02/china-stem-cell/

How Can China Do This?
Science Progress. "China's Recipe for Stem Cell Success."
Accessed February 6, 2013.
http://scienceprogress.org/2010/-02/china-stem-cell/

Didn't That Result in Inferior Medical Practices?
Science Progress. "China's Recipe for Stem Cell Success."
Accessed February 6, 2013.
http://scienceprogress.org/2010/-02/china-stem-cell/

Are Smaller Countries Surpassing the U.S. in Stem Cell Applications?
Science Progress. "China's Recipe for Stem Cell Success."
Accessed February 6, 2013.
http://scienceprogress.org/2010/-02/china-stem-cell/

Chapter 5:

The Importance of Advocates

How Did First Lady Nancy Reagan Become a Believer?
Ronald Reagan Presidential Library and Foundation. "Nancy Reagan: Advocating for Stem Cell Research Post Presidency."
Accessed July 1, 2013.
www.reaganfoundation.org.

ABC News. "Nancy Reagan Pushes for Stem Cell Research."
Accessed Oct. 16, 2012.
http://abcnews.go.com.

Did She Voice Her Support for Stem Cells?
Ronald Reagan Presidential Library and Foundation. "Nancy Reagan: Advocating for Stem Cell Research Post Presidency."
Accessed July 1, 2013.
http://www.reaganfoundation.org.

What has Michael J. Fox Done for Stem Cell Research?
Michael J. Fox Foundation. "Fox Foto Friday: Foundation Awards Over $56 Million to Parkinson's Research in 2012."
Accessed February 4, 2012.
http://www.michaeljfox.org.

Michael J. Fox Foundation. "Stem Cell Board Recommends $14.9 Million for Parkinson's Projects."
Accessed February 4, 2013.
http://www.michaeljfox.org.

Has Fox Supported Embryonic Stem Cell Research?
CNN. "CNN Special: Michael J. Fox talks to Sanjay Gupta."
Accessed February 7, 2013. www.youtube.com/watch?v=la63uShbtsc.

But Hasn't He Since Withdrawn His Support?
Michael J. Fox Foundation. "Stem Cells and Parkinson's Disease: What is the Michael J. Fox Foundation's View on Stem Cells to Treat Parkinson's Disease?"
Accessed February 4, 2013.
https://www.michaeljfox.org/understanding-parkinsons/living-with-pd/topic.php?stem-cells.

Oprah. "Finding a Cure for Parkinson's/Video."
Posted March 31, 2009.
https: www.oprah.com.

And Who is Michael J. Fox?
Michael J. Fox Foundation. "Michael's Story."
Accessed July 1, 2013.
https://www.michaeljfox.org/foundation/michael-story.html.

What Happened to Superman Actor Christopher Reeve?
Christopher & Dana Reeve Foundation. "Christopher Reeve: Biography." Accessed July 1, 2013.
https://Christopherreeve.org.

Why Did He Seek Treatment in Israel?
Israel Ministry of Foreign Affairs. "Christopher Reeve-Caregivers and Scientists are all working with a Sense of Urgency.
Posted July 31, 2003.
http://mfa.gov.il/MFA/PressRoom/2003/Pages/Christopher%20Reeve-%20C aregivers%20and%20scientists%20are%20a.aspx

U.S. News. "Superhero Flies to Israel."
Posted August 3, 2003.
http://www.usnews.com/usnews/news/articles/030811/11spotlight_print.htm.

How Did Reeve Further Early Government Knowledge about Stem Cells?
Christopher Reeve Homepage. "Christopher Reeve Testimony: March 5, 2002." Accessed July 1, 2013.
http://www.chrisreevehomepage.com/sp-testimony-bill1758.html.

NBC News. "California Gives Go-Ahead to Stem-Cell Research."
Accessed July 1, 2013.
http://www.nbcnews.com/id/6384390/ns/health-cloning_and_stem_cells/t/ca lifornia-gives-go-aheadto-stem-cell-research/#.UdIHi_lJOAg.

Have There Been Other Celebrity Endorsers?
Cox News Service (re-post). "Celebrity Spotlight on Stem-Cell Research: Fox, Tyler Moore ask for funds as Critics Cite Moral Objections."
Accessed November 1, 2012.
www.mult-sclerosis.org/news/Sep2000/CelebritiesStemCellResearch.html.

USA Today. "Gov. Schwarzenegger in Tight Political Spot on Stem Cells." Accessed July 2, 2013.
http://usatoday30.usatoday.com/tech/news/techpolicy/2004-08-07-calif-stem cell_x.htm.

Chapter 6:

Therapeutic Advances in Stem Cell Research

What is Stem Cell Replacement Therapy
MichaelJFox.org. "Dr. Lorenz Studer Pioneers Novel Stem Cell Technique in Pre-Clinical Models of Parkinson's Disease."
Accessed February 4, 2013.
https://www.michaeljfox.org/foundation/publication-detail.html?id+103&category=3.

Is This Easy?
MichaelJFox.org. "Dr. Lorenz Studer Pioneers Novel Stem Cell Technique in Pre-Clinical Models of Parkinson's Disease."
Accessed February 4, 2013.
https://www.michaeljfox.org/foundation/publication-detail.html?id+103&category=3.

What Are Clinical Trials?
National Institute of Health. "Learn about Clinical Studies."
Accessed February 4, 2013.
http://clinical trials.gov/ct2/about-studies/learn.

MichaelJFox.org. "How Do We Get Cures?"
Accessed February 4, 2013.
http://www.michaeljfox.org/foundation/news-detail.php?how-do-we-get-cures-clinical-trials .

What Are Double-Blind, Randomized Controlled Trials?
PubMed. "The Double-Blind, Randomized, Placebo-Controlled Trial: Gold Standard or Golden Calf?"
Accessed February 12, 2013.
http://www.ncbi.nlm.nih.gov/pubmed/11377113.

Tony Lu, MD, personal correspondence to Karen McLaren, August 20, 2012.

Tony Lu, MD, personal correspondence to Karen McLaren, August 29, 2012.

What Is Translational Medicine?
Tony Lu, MD, personal correspondence to Karen McLaren, August 28, 2012.

Will Recent Stem Cell Research Change the Way Doctors Treat Disease?
National Institute of Health. "ClinicalTrials.gov: A Service of the U.S. National Institutes of Health."
Accessed November 1, 2012.
http://clinicaltrials.gov/ct2/results?term=stem+cells+&Search+Search.

What Do Researchers Hope to Learn About ...

Aging:

In a study presented at ... The Buck Institute
Genetic and environmental rejuvenation of aging stem cells (Sunday, March 11, 2012) The Buck Institute for Research on Aging held a symposium on Stem Cell Research and Aging March 1-2, 2012 in Novato, California.

They exposed older stem cells
Conboy MJ, et al. "Heterochronic Parabiosis: Historical Perspective and Methodological Considerations for Studies of Aging and Longevity."
Aging Cell. 2013 Jun; 12 (3): 525-30.
doi: 10.1111/acel.12065.Epub 2013 Apr 10.

Villeda, S., et al. "The Ageing Systemic Milieu Negatively Regulates Neurogenesis and Cognitive Function." *Nature* 477 (September 1, 2011); 90-94. doi:10.1038/nature10357.

Incidentally, cosmetic surgeons
Morikuni T, et al. "Adipose-derived Stem Cells: Current Findings and Future Perspectives." *Discovery Medicine*; ISSN: 1539-6509; *Discov Med* 11 (57): 160-170, February 2011.

In humans, innovative cosmetic surgeons are using fat/
Fat grafting offers some benefits ...
Interview with Tony Lu, MD. October 12, 2012.

Nataloni R. "Fat Grafting with Adipocyte Stem Cells Boosts Facial Volume." Cosmetic Surgery Times (May 1, 2010).
Accessed September, 27, 2012.
http://cosmeticsurgerytimes.modernmedicine.com.

Cohen SR, et al. "Adipocyte-derived Stem and Regenerative Cells in Facial Rejuvenation." *Clin Plast Surg.* 2012 Oct; 39 (4): 453-64.
doi: 10.1016/j.cps.2012.07.014.

Lam SM. "Fat Grafting: An Alternative or Adjunct to Facelift Surgery?" *Facial Plast Surg Clin North Am.* 2013 May; 21 (2): 253-64.
doi: 10.1016/j.fsc.2013.02.005.

ALS (Lou Gehrig's Disease):

Are Clinical Trials Making the Progression

Informa Health Care. "Mesenchymal Stromal Cells Prolong the Lifespan in a Rat Model of Amyotrophic Lateral Sclerosis."
Accessed May 11, 2013.
http://informahealthcare.com/doi/abs/10.3109/14653249.2011.592521.

Liebert Online. "Intracerebroventricular Administration of Human Umbilical Cord Blood Cells Delays Disease Progression in Two Murine Models of Motor Neuron Degeneration."
Accessed May11, 2013.
http://www.liebertonline.com/doi/abs/10.1089/rej.2011.1197.

www.neuralstem.com/cell-therapy-for-als. Accessed August 12, 2013.

Also worth reading:

Mazzini L, et al. "Mesenchymal Stem Cell Transplantation in Amyotrophic Lateral Sclerosis: A Phase I Clinical Trial." *Exp Neurol.* 2010 May; 223 (1): 229-37.
doi: 10.1016/j.expneurol.2009. 08.007.Epub 2009 Aug 13.
http://www.sciencedirect.com/science/article/pii/S0014488609003173.

Mazzini L, et al. "Mesenchymal Stromal Cell Transplantation in Amyotrophic Lateral Sclerosis: A Long-term Safety Study." *Cytotherapy.* 2012 Jan; 14 (1): 56-60.
doi:10.3109/14653249.2011.613929. Epub 2011 Sep 28.
http://informahealthcare.com/doi/abs/10.3109/14653249.2011.613929.

Soler B, et al. "Stem Cells Therapy in Amyotrophic Lateral Sclerosis Treatment. A Critical View."
Rev Neurol. 2011 Apr 1; 52 (7): 426-34.
http://www.ncbi.nlm.nih.gov/pubmed/21425112.

Springer Link. "Stem Cell Transplantation for Motor Neuron Disease: Current Approaches and Future Perspectives."
Accessed May 12, 2013.
http://www.springerlink.com/content/h7r7783452420177/

Future Medicine. "Stem Cell Technology for the Study and Treatment of Motor Neuron Diseases."
Accessed May 12,2013.
http://www.futuremedicine.com/doi/abs/10.2217/rme.11.6?journalCode=rme.

Alzheimer's Disease:

What are Potential Keys to Eliminating Alzheimer's

Sugaya, Kiminobu. "Possible Use of Autologous Stem Cell Therapies for Alzheimer's Disease." *Curr Alzheimer Res.* 2005 Jul; 2(3): 367-76.

Nevertheless, human neural stem cells

Jin K, et al. "Delayed Transplantation of Human Neural Precursor Cells Improves Outcome from Focal Cerebral Ischemia in Aged Rats."
Aging Cell. 2010 Dec; 9 (6): 1076-83.
doi: 10.1111/j.1474-9726.2010.00638.x.

Wislet-Gendebien S, et al. "Mesenchymal Stem Cells and Neural Crest Cells from Adult Bone Marrow: Characterization of their Surprising Similarities and Differences." *Cell Mol Life Sci.* 2012 Aug; 69 (15): 2593-608.
doi: 10.1007/s00018-012-0937-1. Epub 2012 Feb 19.

Researchers are also questioning glia's role

Sugaya K., et al. "Stem Cell Strategies for Alzheimer's Disease Therapy." *Panminerva Medica* 2006 Jun; 48(2):87-96.

Also worth reading :

Sugaya K, et al. "How to Approach Alzheimer's Disease Therapy Using Stem Cell Technologies". *J Alzheimers Dis.* 2008 Oct; 15 (2): 241-54.

Singh S, et al. "Current Therapeutic Strategy in Alzheimer's Disease". *Eur Rev Med Pharmacol Sci.* 2012 Nov; 16 (12): 1651-64.

Gonzalez-Castaneda RE, et al. "Neurogenesis in Alzheimer's Disease: A Realistic Alternative to Neuronal Degeneration?" *Curr Signal Transduct Ther.* 2011 Sep 1; 6(3): 314-319.

Autism:

Does Hope Lie in Stem Cells

Ichim TE, et al. "Stem Cell Therapy for Autism". *J Transl Med.* 2007 Jun 27; 5:30.

In August 2012,
Craft CH. "Neuroscience Institute Launching Trial of Cord Blood Stem Cells in Autistic Children." *The Sacramento Bee.*
Published Tuesday, Aug 21, 2012 - 12:00 am/page 1A.

Favorable results have been documented

Siniscalco D, et al. "Autism Spectrum Disorders: Is Mesenchymal Stem Cell Personalized Therapy the Future?" *J Biomed Biotechnol.* 2012; 2012: 480289.
doi: 10. 1155/2012/480289. Epub 2012 Feb 13.

Translational Medicine. "Stem Cell Treatment Doing Wonders for Autistic Glenburn Boy."
Posted June 25, 2010.
http://www.translational-medicine.com/content/5/1/30/abstract.

http://www.wabi.tv/news/7451/glenburn-boy-returns-from-costa-rica-after-having-adult-stem-cell-therapy.
Accessed August 11, 2013.

Autoimmune Diseases:

Tyndall, Alan. "Successes and Failures of Stem Cell Transplantation in Autoimmune Diseases."
Hematology Am Soc Hematol Educ Program 2011; 2011: 280-4.
doi: 10.1182/asheducation 2011.1.280.

Bone Marrow Transplants:

Martin D. "Dr. Georges Mathe, Transplant Pioneer Dies at 88."
The New York *Times*.
Published Oct 20, 2010. Accessed Aug 11, 2013.

Cancer:

What New Paths of Discovery

California Institute for Regenerative Medicine. "Genetic Enhancement of the Immune Response to Melanoma via hESC-derived T cells."
http://www.cirm.ca.gov retrieved March 26, 2013.

In order for healthy human immune systems to work

Mantia-Smaldone GM, et al. "A Review of Dendritic Cell Therapy for Cancer: Progress and Challenges." *BioDrugs*. 2013 Apr 17.
[Epub ahead of print]

Galluzzi L, et al. "Trial Watch: Dendritic Cell-based Interventions for Cancer Therapy." *Oncoimmunology*. 2012 Oct 1; 1 (7): 1111-1134.

The delicate equilibrium
www.cirm.ca.gov/node/9595/review.
Accessed August 12, 2013.

Researchers in Singapore

Kandasamy M, et al. "Complement Mediated Signaling on Pulmonary CD 103+ Dendritic Cells is Critical for their Migratory Function in Response to Influenza Infection. *PLos Pathog* 9 (1): e1003115.
doi: 10.1371/journal.ppat.1003115.

Horden A O, et al. "The First Dendritic Cell-based Therapeutic Cancer Vaccine is Approved by the FDA." *Scandinavian Journal of Immunology*, 72: 554.
doi: 10.1111/j.1365-3083.2010.02464x.

Also worth reading:

Berinstein, Neil L. et al. "First-in-man Application of a Novel Therapeutic Cancer Vaccine Formulation with the Capacity to Induce Multi-functional T Cell Responses in Ovarian, Breast and Prostate Cancer Patients." *Journal of Translational Medicine* 10 (2012); 156.
doi: 10.1186/1479-5876-10-156.

Azvolinsky A. "One Size Does Not Fit All: Personalized Immune Therapies Poised to Take Center Stage." *J Natl Cancer Inst.* 2013 May 1; 105 (9): 583-4.
doi: 10.1093/jnci/djt 103. Epub 2013 Apr 16.

www.fda.gov/BiologicBloodVaccines/CellularGeneTherapyProducts/Ap provedProducts/default.htm.
Accessed August 11, 2013.

Scientists at the University of Michigan

www.cancer.med.umich.edu/research/breast_stemcells_two.shtml.
Accessed August 12, 2013.

www.cirm.ca.gov/node/9595/review.
Accessed August 12, 2013.

More than a dozen years after experimental treatment

www.cirmresearch.blogspot.com/2011/07/aggressive-breast-cancer-trea
ted-with.html (July 25, 2011: Aggressive breast cancer treated with bone
marrow stem cells).
Accessed August 11, 2013.

med.stanford.edu/ism/2011/july/breast-cancer.html.
Accessed Aug 8, 2013.

Also worth reading:

www.cirm.ca.gov/about-stem-cells/malignant-glioma-fact-sheet.
Accessed March 26, 2013.

Standard (cytotoxic) chemotherapy

Marsh JC, et al. "Current Status of Immunotherapy and Gene Therapy for
High-grade Gliomas." *Cancer Control*. 2013 Jan; 20 (1): 43-8.

Gursel DB, et al. "Trials and Tribulations of Cancer Immunotherapy: The
Dendritic Cell Vaccine Shows Promise in a Phase I Glioblastoma
Multiforme Trial." *Neurosurgery*. 2012 Dec; 71 (6): N19-21.
doi: 10.1227/01.neu.0000423045.97311.f7.

Cerebral Palsy:

Are Therapies Showing Promise

Kirby RS, et al. "Prevalence and Functioning of Children with Cerebral
Palsy in Four Areas of the United States in 2006: A Report from the
Autism and Developmental Disabilities Monitoring Network." *Res Dev
Disabil*. 2011 Mar-Apr; 32 (2): 462-9. Epub 2011 Jan 26.

Uchida N, et al. "Human Neural Stem Cells Induce Functional
Myelination in Mice with Severe Dysmyelination. *Sci Transl Med* 4 (155):
155ra136.
doi: 10.1126/scitranslmed.3004371PMID: 23052293.

In a human trial, researchers injected stem cells

Li, Min. "Treatment of One Case of Cerebral Palsy Combined with Posterior Visual Pathway Injury Using Autologous Bone Marrow Mesenchymal Stem Cells." *Journal of Translational Medicine* 10 (2012): 100.
doi: 10.1186/1479-5876-10-100.

Chaitanya P, et al. "Therapeutic Potential of Autologous Stem Cell Transplantation for Cerebral Palsy." *Case Reports in Transplantation.* Volume 2012 (2012), Article ID 825289, 6 pages.
http://dx.doi.org/10.1155/2012/825289.

Still in other research

Lee YH, et al. "Safety and Feasibility of Countering Neurological Impairment by Intravenous Administration of Autologous Cord Blood in Cerebral Palsy." *Journal of Translational Medicine* 10 (2012):58.
doi: 10.1186/1479-5876-10-58.

Also worth reading:

http://www.ninds.nih.gov/disorders/cerebral_palsy/detail_cerebral_palsy.htm.
Accessed Aug 8, 2013.

Diabetes:

While researchers have shown

Schultz, TC et al. "A Scalable System for Production of Functional Pancreatic Progenitors from Human Embryonic Stem Cells." *PLoS One.* 2012; 7 (5): e37004.
doi: 10.1371/journal.pone.0037004. Epub 2012 May 18.

Meanwhile in Brussels

Grouwels, G. et al. "Differentiating Neural Crest Stem Cells Induce Proliferation of Cultured Rodent Islet Beta Cells." *Diabetologia.* 2012 Jul; 55 (7): 2016-25.
doi: 10.1007/s00125-012-2542-0. Epub 2012 May 23.

In Israel

Fishman B, et al. "Targeting Pancreatic Progenitor Cells in Human Embryonic Stem Cell Differentiation for the Identification of Novel Cell Surface Markers." *Stem Cell Rev.* 2012 Sep; 8 (3): 792-802.
doi: 10.1007/s12015-012-9363-x.

Even researchers in India

Joglekar, MV and Hardikar, AA. "Isolation, Expansion, and Characterization of Human Islet-derived Progenitor Cells." *Methods Mol Biol.* 2012; 879: 351-66.
doi: 10 1007/978-1-61779-815-3_21.

Other studies hope to cure

Si, Y. et al. "Infusion of Mesenchymal Stem Cells Ameliorates Hyperglycemia in Type 2 Diabetic Rats: Identification of a Novel Role in Improving Insulin Sensitivity." *Diabetes.* 2012 Jun; 61 (6): 1616-25.
doi: 10.2337/db11-1141.

Mesenchymal stem cells in human umbilical cord

Kadam, S. et al. "Generation of Functional Islets from Human Umbilical Cord and Placenta Derived Mesenchymal Stem Cells." *Methods Mol Biol.* 2012; 879: 291-313.
doi: 10.1007/978-1-61779-815-3_17.

Also worth reading:

Gitelman SE, et al. "Autologous Nonmyeloablative Hematopoietic Stem Cell Transplantation in Newly Diagnosed Type 1 Diabetes Mellitus." *JAMA.* 2009 Aug 12; 302 (6): 624; author reply 624-5.
doi: 10.1001/jama.2009.1098.
http://jama.ama-assn.org/content/297/14/1568.short.

Jurewicz M, et al. "Congenic Mesenchymal Stem Cell Therapy Reverses Hyperglycemia in Experimental Type 1 Diabetes." *Diabetes.* 2010 Dec; 59 (12): 3139-47.
doi: 10.2337/DB 10-0542. Epub 2010 Sep 14.
http://diabetes.diabetesjournals.org/content/59/12/3139.short.

Aguayo-Mazzucato C, et al. "Stem Cell Therapy for Type 1 Diabetes Mellitus." *Nat Rev Endocrinol.* 2010 Mar; 6 (3): 139-48.
doi: 10.1038/nrendo.2009.274.

Mabed M, et al. "Mesenchymal Stem Cell-based Therapy for the Treatment of Type 1 Diabetes Mellitus". *Curr Stem Cell Res Ther.* 2012 May; 7 (3): 179-90.

Emphysema (COPD; Respiratory Diseases):
Chronic obstructive pulmonary disease (COPD), occurs

Barbera, J.A. and Peinado, V.I. "Vascular Progenitor Cells in Chronic Obstructive Pulmonary Disease." Department of Pulmonary Medicine, Hospital Clinic, Universitat de Barcelona, Barcelona, Spain.
Jbarbera@clinic.ub.es.

Therefore, stem cell regeneration is a promising solution

Kubo H. "Regenerative Approach for COPD." *Nihon Rinsho.* 2011 Oct; 69 (10): 1869-72. Article in Japanese.

It should be noted that some Italian researchers

Caramori, G., et al. "Role of Stem Cells in the Pathogenesis of Chronic Obstructive Pulmonary Disease and of Pulmonary Emphysema." Dipartimento di Medicina, Universita di Ferrara, Italy. Gaetano.caramori@unife.it.

There is evidence in mice

Xian, W. and McKeon, F. "Adult Stem Cells Underlying Lung Regeneration." Institute of Medical Biology; A-STAR; Singapore and Department of Pathology; Brigham and Women's Hospital; Boston, MA USA.

Meanwhile, mesenchymal Stem Cell therapy
Jungebluth, P. et al. "Mesenchymal Stem Cells Restore Lung Function by Recruiting Resident and Non-resident Proteins."

Other studies have confirmed

Abreu, S.C. et al. "Mechanisms of Cellular Therapy in Respiratory Diseases." Laboratorio de Investigacao Pulmonar, Centro de Ciencias da Saude, Instituto de Biofisica Carlos Chagas Filho, Universidade Federal do Rio de Janeiro, Avenida Carlos Chagas Filho.

Heart Attacks & Heart Damage:

Are Small Steps Laying the Foundation

Raj MR, et al. "Intracoronary Cardiosphere-derived Cells for Heart Regeneration after Myocardial Infarction (CADUCEUS): A Prospective, Randomized Phase 1 Trial." *Lancet.* 2012 March; 379 (9819): 895-904. doi: 10.1016/S0140-6736 (12) 60195-0.

When a company employs researchers

Athena Trial using adipose-derived regenerative cells to treat chronic heart failure from coronary heart disease. Clinicaltrials.gov (NCT01556022).
Accessed August 12, 2013.
www.theathenatrial.com

Also worth reading:

Bolli R, et al. "Cardiac Stem Cell in Patients with Ischaemic Cardiomyopathy (SCIPIO): Initial Results of a Randomized Phase 1 Trial." *Lancet.* 2011 November; 378 (9806): 1847-1857. doi: 10.1016/S0140-6736 (11) 61590-0.

Hamano K, et al. "Local Implantation of Autologous Bone Marrow Cells for Therapeutic Angiogenesis in Patients with Ischaemic Heart Disease: Clinical Trial and Preliminary Results." *Jpn Circ J.* 2001 Sep; 65 (9): 845-7.

Strauer BE, et al. "Repair of Infarcted Myocardium by Autologous Intracoronary Mononuclear Bone Marrow Cell Transplantation in Humans." *Circulation.* 2002; 106: 1913-18.

Assmus B, et al. "Transplantation of Progenitor Cells and Regeneration Enhancement in Acute Myocardial Infarction." *Circulation.* 2002 Dec 10; 106 (24): 3009-17.

Fuchs S, et al. "Safety and Feasibility of Transendocardial Autologous Bone Marrow Cell Transplantation in Patients with Advanced Heart Disease." *Am J Cardiol.* 2006 Mar 15; 97 (6): 823-9. Epub 2006 Jan 30.

Fuchs S, et al. "Catheter-based Autologous Bone Marrow Myocardial Injection in No-option Patients with Advanced CoronaryAartery Disease: A Feasibility Study." *J Am Coll Cardiol.* 2003 May 21; 41 (10): 1721-4.

Perin EC, et al. "Transendocardial, Autologous Bone Marrow Cell Transplantation for Severe, Chronic Ischemic Heart Failure." *Circulation.* 2003 May 13; 107 (18): 2294-302. Epub 2003 Apr 21.

Tse HF, et al. "Angiogenesis in Ischemic Myocardium by Intramyocardial Autologous Bone Marrow Mononuclear Cell Implantation." *Lancet.* 2003 Jan 4; 361 (9351): 47-9.

Stamm C, et al. "Autologous Bone Marrow Stem Cell Transplantation for Myocardial Regeneration." *Lancet.* 2003 Jan 4; 361 (9351): 45-6.

Clifford DM, et al. "Stem Cell Treatment for Acute Myocardial Infarction." *Cochrane Database Syst Rev.* 2012 Feb 15; 2: CD006536. doi: 10.1002/14651858.CD006536.pub2.

Wollert KC, et al. "Intracoronary Autologous Bone Marrow Cell Transfer after Myocardial Infarction: The BOOST Randomized Controlled Clinical Trial." *Lancet.* 2004 Jul 10-16; 364 (9429): 141-8.

Stamm C, et al. "CABG and Bone Marrow Stem Cell Transplantation after Myocardial Infarction. *J Thorac Cardiovasc Surg.* 2004 Jun; 52 (3): 152-8.

HIV:

A 45-year old man known as 'the Berlin Patient'

Allers K et al. "Evidence for the Cure of HIV Infection by CCR5?32/ ?32 Stem Cell Transplantation." *Blood.* 2011 Mar 10; 117 (10): 2791-9. doi: 10.1182/blood-2010-09-309591. Epub 2010 Dec 8.

Petz LD, et al. "Hematopoietic Cell Transplantation with Cord Blood for Cure of HIV Infections." *Biol Blood MarrowTransplant.* 2013 Mar; 19 (3): 393-7.
doi: 10.1016/j.bbmt. 2012.10.017. Epub 2012 Oct 23.

Clearly, this case showed that bone marrow transplants

http://abcnews.go.com 'Berlin Patient' Timothy Brown Says He is Still HIV-Free, Lisa Mcclellan, M.D. July 24, 2012.
Accessed April 12, 2013.

Liver Damage:

Takanori T, et al. "Vascularized and Functional Human Liver From an iPSC-derived Organ Bud Transplant." *Nature* (2013). Published online 03 July 2013. doi: 10.1038/nature12271.
www-user.yokohama-cu.ac.jp/-saisei/
Accessed Aug 15, 2013.

Also worth reading:

Yu Wang, et al. "Adipose Derived Mesenchymal Stem Cells Transplantation via Portal Vein Improves Microcirculation and Ameliorates Liver Fibrosis Induced by CCl4 in Rats." *Journal of Translational Medicine.* 2012, 10: 133.
doi: 10.1186/1479-5876-10-133.

Drosos I, et al. "Stem Cells in Liver Regeneration and Their Potential Clinical Applications." *Stem Cell Rev.* 2013 Mar 24.

Seki A, et al. "Adipose Tissue-derived Stem Cell as a Regenerative Therapy for a Murine Steatohepatitis-induced Cirrhosis Model." *Hepatology.* 2013 May 17.
doi: 10.1002/hep.26470.

Macular Degeneration:

Scientists have injected

Schwartz SD, et al. "Embryonic Stem Cell Trial for Macular Degeneration: A Preliminary Report."
www.thelancet.com. Published online January 23, 2012.
doi: 10.1016/S0140-6736(12)60028-2.

Additionally, Japanese researchers

Scicasts.com/stem-cells/6366-pilot-clinical-study-into-ips-cell-therapy-for-eye-disease-starts-in-japan.

Also worth reading:

Wong I Y, et al. "Promises of Stem Cell Therapy for Retinal Degenerative Diseases." *Graefes Arch Clin Exp Ophthalmol.* 2011 Oct; 249 (10): 1439-48.
doi: 10.1007/s00417-1764-z. Epub 2011 Aug 25.

Ramsden C M, et al. "Stem Cells in Retinal Regeneration: Past, Present and Future." *Development.* 2013 Jun; 140 (12): 2576-85.
doi: 10.1242/dev.092270.

Pan C K, et al. "Embryonic Stem Cells as a Treatment for Macular Degeneration." *Expert Opin Biol Ther.* 2013 Aug; 13 (8): 1125-33. doi: 10.1517/14712598.2013.793304. Epub 2013 May 25.

Multiple Sclerosis (MS):

The Cleveland Clinic has begun

Cleveland.com Northeast Ohio. "Clinical Trials Using Adult Stem Cells to Treat MS." Updated August 24, 2011.
Accessed April 9, 2013.
http://www.cleveland.com/healthfit/index.ssf/2011/08/cleveland_clinic_uh_a nd_cwru_c.html

my.clevelandclinic.org/media_relations/library/2011/2011-08-23-cleveland-r esearchers-collaborate-to-launch-phase-1-clinical-trial-for-new-multiple-scler osis-treatment.aspx.

Paddock C. "Major International Stem Cell Trials for Multiple Sclerosis Get Funding." Medical News Today. *MediLexicon, Intl.*, 30 Jul. 2011. Web. 12 Aug. 2013.
Accessed August 12, 2013.
http://www.medicalnewstoday.com/articles/231944.php.

Also worth reading:

Payne N, et al. "The Prospect of Stem Cells as Multi-faceted Purveyors of Immune Modulation, Repair and Regeneration in Multiple Sclerosis." Curr Stem *Cell Res Ther.* 2011 Mar; 6 (1): 50-62.

Slavin S, et al. "The Potential Use of Adult Stem Cells for the Treatment of Multiple Sclerosis and Other Neurodegenerative Disorders." *Clin Neurol Neurosurg.* 2008 Nov; 110 (9): 943-6.
doi: 10.1016/j. clineuro.2008.01.014. Epub 2008 Mar 6.

Muscular Dystrophy:

Treatment for muscular dystrophy has been hampered

Filareto A, et al. "An Ex Vivo Gene Therapy Approach to Treat Muscular Dystrophy Using Inducible Pluripotent Stem Cells." *Nature Communications.* 2013; 4 (1549).
doi: 10.1038/ncomms2550.

In addition, researchers at Purdue University

Liu WY, et al. "Hypoxia Promotes Satellite Cell Self-renewal and Enhances the Efficiency of Myoblast Transplantation." *Development.* 2012 Aug; 139: 2857-2865.
doi: 10.1242/dev.079665.

Children with the specific form of Duchenne

Conger K. "New Mouse Model Reveals a Mystery of Duchenne Muscular Dystrophy, Scientists Report." *Stanford School of Medicine News.* July 7, 2013.
Accessed August 15, 2013.
Med.stanford.edu/ism/2013/july/blau.html.

Also worth reading:

Kocaefe C, et al. "Reprogramming of Human Umbilical Cord Stromal Mesenchymal Stem Cells for Myogenic Differentiation and Muscle Repair." *Stem Cell Rev.* 2010 Dec; 6 (4): 512-22.
doi: 10.1007/s12015-010-9177-7.

Meng J, et al. "Stem Cells to Treat Muscular Dystrophies - Where Are We?" *Neuromuscul Disord.* 2011 Jan; 21 (1): 4-12.
doi: 10.1016/j.nmd.2010.10.004. Epub 2010 Nov 4.

Negroni E, et al. "Current Advances in Cell Therapy Strategies for Muscular Dystrophies." *Expert Opin Biol Ther.* 2011 Feb; 11 (2): 157-76.
doi: 10.1517/14712598.2011.542748.

Osteoarthritis & Osteoporosis:

Repairing a bone fracture or replacing a hip

Science 20. "Degradable Plastic Implants and Adult Stem Cells Make Light Work of Broken Bones."
Accessed February 13, 2013.
htpp://www.science20.com/news_articles/degradable_plastic_implants_and_adult_stem_ce.

Researchers theorize that

University of Southampton. "News Release: Stem Cell Breakthrough Could Lead to New Bone Repair Therapies on Nanoscale Surfaces."
Ref: 13/27.
Accessed February 13, 2013.
http://southhampton.ac.uk/mediacenter/news/2013/feb/13_27.shtml.

University of Glasgow. "Research and Innovation: The Future of Fracture Fixing."
Accessed February 13, 2013.
http://gla.ac.uk/research/keyresearchareas/interdisciplinaryresearch/nanotechnology/

In a related study in Malaysia

Saw KY, et al. "Articular Cartilage Regeneration with Autologous Peripheral Blood Progenitor Cells and Hyaluronic Acid after Arthroscopic Subchondral Drilling: A Report of 5 Cases with Histology. *Arthroscopy: The Journal of Arthroscopic and Related Surgery.* 2011 April; 27 (4): 493-506.

Parkinson's Disease:

Doctors already know that a specific type

EuroStemCell. "Parkinson's disease: how could stem cells help?"
Last updated March 16, 2012. Accessed August 16, 2012.
http://www.eurostemcell.org/factsheet/parkinson's-disease-how-could-stem-cells-help .

Furthermore, at the Buck Institute for Research

Kordower JH, et al. "Lewy Body-like Pathology in Long-term Embryonic Nigral Transplants in Parkinson's Disease." *Nature Medicine* 2008, 14 (5): 504-506.

Also worth reading:

Ali F, et al. "Stem Cells and the Treatment of Parkinson's Disease." *Exp Neurol.* 2013 Jan 6. Pii: S0014-4886 (13) 00004-6. doi: 10.1016/j.expneurol. 2012. 12.017.

Orlacchio A, et al. "Stem Cells: An Overview of the Current Status of Therapies for Central and Peripheral Nervous System Diseases." *Curr Med Chem.* 2010; 17 (7): 595-608.

Spinal Cord Injury:

Early findings in a randomized trial

Elkheir WA, et al. "Autologous Bone Marrow-derived Stem Cell Therapy Combined with Physical Therapy Induces Functional Improvement in Chronic Spinal Cord Injury Patients." *Cell Transplantation.* April 12, 2013. doi: http://dx.doi.org/10.3727/096368913X664540.

A small trial at the Spinal Cord Injury Center

StemCells, Inc. "StemCells, Inc. Reports Positive Interim Data From Spinal Cord Injury Trial."
Accessed April 2, 2013.
http://investor.stemcellsinc.com/phoenix.zhtml.

Also worth reading:

Science Daily. "New Hope for Reversing the Effects of Spinal Cord Injury." Posted March 12, 2013.
Accessed March 31, 2013.
http://www.sciencedaily.com/releases/2013/03/130312151947.htm.

http://investor.stemcellsinc.conm/phoenix.zhtml?c=86230&p=irol-ne
wsArticle&ID=1730805 ... StemCells, Inc. Reports Positive Interim Data
From Spinal Cord Injury Trial Sept. 3, 2012 (GlobeNewswire).
Accessed April 4, 2013.

Park DH, et al. "Transplantation of Umbilical Cord Blood Stem Cells for
Treating Spinal Cord Injury." *Stem Cell Rev.* 2011 Mar; 7 (1): 181-94.
doi: 10.1007/s12015-010-9163-0.

Li J, et al. "Cell Transplantation for Spinal Cord Injury: A Systematic
Review." *Biomed Res Int.* 2013: 786475.
doi: 10.1155/2013/786475. Epub 2013 Jan 15.

Stroke:

In more than 80% of strokes

Saver JL. "Time is Brain - Quantified". *Stroke.* 2006; 37: 263-266.
doi: 10.1161/01.STR.0000196957.55928.ab.

Researchers are experimenting with

Advance for Physical Therapy & Rehab Medicine. "News and Notes:
Researchers Study Stem Cell Therapy for Stroke."
Accessed March 29, 2013.
http//physical-therapy.advanceweb.com.

In Glasgow, a small study

Paddock C. "Stroke Patients Show Signs of Recovery Following Stem Cell
Trial". *Medical News Today* 28 May, 2013 (Updated interim results of the
Pilot Investigation of Stem Cells in Stroke PISCES Trial).
Accessed August 14, 2013.
www.medicalnewstoday.com/article/261084.php.

Also worth reading:

Locatelli F, et al. "Stem Cell Therapy in Stroke." *Cell Mol Life Sci.* 2009
Mar; 66 (5): 757-72.
doi: 10.1007/s00018-008-8346-1.

Yu F, et al. "Adult Stem Cells and Bioengineering Strategies for the Treatment of Cerebral Ischemic Stroke." *Curr Stem Cell Res Ther.* 2011 Sep; 6 (3): 190-207.

Lee JS, et al. "A Long-term Follow-up Study of Intravenous Autologous Mesenchymal Stem Cell Transplantation in Patients with Ischemic Stroke." *Stem Cells.* 2010 Jun; 28 (6): 1099-106.
doi: 10.1002/stem.430.

www.telegraph.co.uk/science/science-news/9333185/Stem-cell-treatment-helps-heal. Stem Cell Treatment Helps Heal Stroke Victims
posted June 15, 2012.
Accessed March 31, 2013.

About the Author

TONY LU, M.D., M.B.A.

Tony Lu has the microscopic eye of a bench scientist and the insight of a physician who has seen the world through many diverse cultures and cities. Born of Chinese descent, he immigrated to the United States and became a United States citizen along the way to a medical career that has spanned three decades. He has practiced in outstanding hospitals and clinics from New York, to Chicago and Seattle.

Most recently he served as the Chief Medical Officer at WA Regenerative Medicine, Ltd. in Shanghai, China; and at United Family Healthcare in Guangzhou, China. This is where his interest in stem cell medicine escalated, where he witnessed his Asian colleagues making significant findings that were encouraged there, but are not possible yet in the United States. He wanted so much to be a part of this new medical frontier!

Dr. Lu has comprehensive working knowledge of East meets West integrated medicine, including both functional and regenerative aspects of treatment. In addition to adult healthcare, he is also proficient in anti-aging, stem cell medicine and medical acupuncture.

Currently Tony Lu is Medical Director for Humana Military Healthcare Services at one of the VA Community Based Outpatient Centers in Seattle, Washington. He is honored to serve returning Veterans from Iraq and Afghanistan, as well as those who were deployed to Vietnam and Korea.

He is a doctor of the world. Tony Lu speaks English, Mandarin, Cantonese, French, and Vietnamese. He admits that beyond communicating primarily in English, "I pray in French, calculate in French, and hold my deepest emotions in Cantonese."

KAREN MCLAREN

Karen McLaren is one of the most fluent writers in healthcare today. For nearly all of her adult life, she has been married to one of the world's longest surviving 'medical miracles', a ground-breaking pioneer of Johns Hopkins Blue Baby life-saving pediatric heart surgery. If life was going to take her into the prestigious world of elite doctors and hospitals, she reasoned, then she would learn as much about as many diseases as possible. Life is precious and she understands what it means to be waiting (anxiously!) for the next advancement with the potential to extend a life. She has witnessed the courage of patients attempting to undergo rare and risky life-saving surgery — and she understands the physical, mental, and emotional toll this takes on both the patient and the patient's family. Physicians and hospitals too are courageous in these endeavors. Every day, in spite of the incredible risks to their own circumstances, they go to work saving lives, easing pain, and discovering better ways to help their patients live.

Professionally, Karen McLaren is president of a boutique advertising agency, specializing in marketing for physicians, hospitals, and other professionals. In her free time, she writes magazine articles — and she is published regularly.

www.ingramcontent.com/pod-product-compliance
Lightning Source LLC
Chambersburg PA
CBHW020157200326
41521CB00006B/409